Me Before/ Me After

Me Before/Me After is a complete programme for professionals who run rehabilitation groups for brain injury survivors. The programme's overarching goal is to retrieve the person behind the injury by helping survivors master the consequences of their brain injury. The approach combines CBT principles that develop awareness and recognition of mental events with CBT techniques that are instrumental in achieving behaviour change. The manual focuses on the three aspects of acquired brain injury that are integral to achieving gains through rehabilitation:

1 Change awareness: develops awareness of the changes that are consequent upon brain injury.
2 Change investigation: helps understand why these changes occur, how we interpret them and how we cope with them.
3 Change mastery: helps gain mastery over these changes by developing and mobilising adaptive capability.

This comprehensive manual includes extensive resources for practitioners, clients and support workers and provides everything you need in order to run the most effective brain injury rehabilitation groups in one place.

Leyla Ziyal is an HCPC registered Chartered Consultant Clinical Neuropsychologist with many years' experience in clinical psychology, neuropsychology, psychological therapies and business psychology.

T0132706

Me Before/ Me After

A Group Rehabilitation Programme for Brain Injury Survivors

Leyla Ziyal

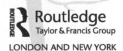

Routledge
Taylor & Francis Group

LONDON AND NEW YORK

First published 2018
by Routledge
2 Park Square, Milton Park, Abingdon, Oxon OX14 4RN

and by Routledge
711 Third Avenue, New York, NY 10017

Routledge is an imprint of the Taylor & Francis Group, an informa business

British Library Cataloguing-in-Publication Data
A catalogue record for this book is available from the British Library

Library of Congress Cataloging-in-Publication Data
Names: Ziyal, Leyla, author.
Title: Me before/me after : a group rehabilitation programme for brain injury
    survivors / Leyla Ziyal.
Description: Milton Park, Abingdon, Oxon ; New York, NY : Routledge, 2018. |
    Includes bibliographical references.
Identifiers: LCCN 2017004196 | ISBN 9781138041967 (hbk) | ISBN
    9781911186045 (pbk) | ISBN 9781315174129 (ebk)
Subjects: LCSH: Brain damage—Patients—Rehabilitation. | Group psychotherapy.
Classification: LCC RC387.5 .Z59 2018 | DDC 617.4/810443—dc23
LC record available at https://lccn.loc.gov/2017004196

ISBN: 978-1-911186-04-5 (pbk)
ISBN: 978-1-315-17412-9 (ebk)

Typeset in NewsGothic BT
by Apex CoVantage, LLC

Visit the eResources: www.routledge.com/9781911186045

MIX
Paper from
responsible sources
FSC
www.fsc.org   FSC® C011748

Contents

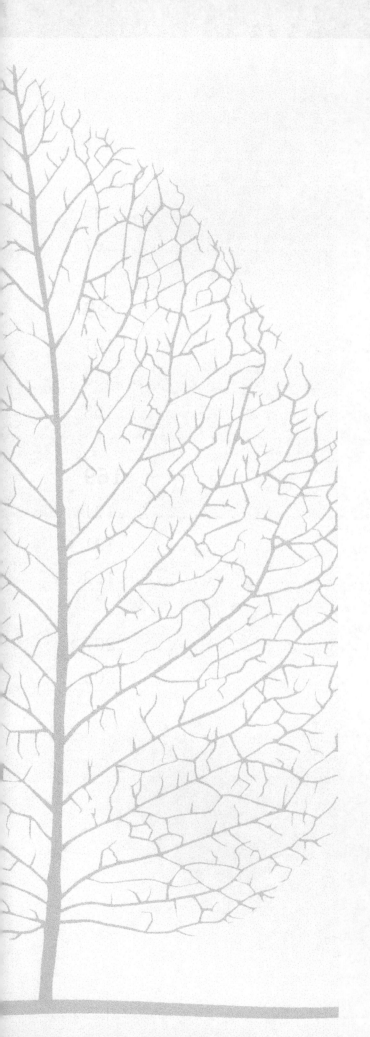

1 Introduction

1.1 Description

This manual is a practical resource for rehabilitation professionals on running a group programme for brain injury survivors. The intervention sits within the cognitive behaviour therapy framework and combines CBT principles that develop awareness and identification of mental events with CBT techniques that are instrumental in achieving behaviour change. The manual is in three modules, focussing on the three aspects of acquired brain injury that are integral to achieving gains through rehabilitation. These are change recognition, change exploration and change mastery.

- **Module 1: Change-Recognition:** Survivors of acquired brain injury (ABI) respond to the onset of impairment with feelings of inferiority, anxiety, loss of confidence, anger and sadness fuelled by unfavourable comparisons between their pre- and post-ABI self-perceptions. They slip into a state of learned helplessness in which they deny, overlook and attempt to hide their disabilities from others and from themselves. This module gently steers participants towards awareness of these changes, towards an understanding of why they have occurred and towards making active decisions on how to deal with them.
- **Module 2: Change-Exploration:** delves into the ways in which the group has been coping with the adverse post-ABI changes that have impacted their day-to-day lives. It is a preparation for partaking in therapy and raises motivation to trial different and adaptive adjustment strategies.
- **Module 3: Change Mastery:** actively engages in therapy with the application of imaginary and real-life exposure to

critical events. Its overarching aim is to enable the group to reconnect with the various contexts in which they live, relate and work, by developing a sense of self-efficacy and direction over events which until then seemed to be beyond their control.

These three modules are anchored to the three key stakeholders of the programme who are Practitioners, Support Workers and Group participants.

- **Practitioners** are the professionals engaged in delivery of the programme. They are post-qualified, experienced ABI rehabilitation professionals who have a good working knowledge of the theory and practice of cognitive behaviour therapy and of running groups. They would be clinical neuropsychologists, occupational therapists, psychiatrists and other mental health practitioners. They provide the programme's continuity and consistency and the achievement of a positive outcome depends on their commitment, skills and effectiveness.
- **Support Workers** are the key resource of the programme. They could be members of any discipline of the interdisciplinary team and have a very important role to play. They are especially assigned to the programme, take part in group sessions and facilitate the subsequent assignment meetings in which they support participants in completing their weekly homework. They know the participants well and in both sessions and meetings they function as auxiliary group therapists.[1] They review and clarify the events of the preceding session and give guidance on how to complete

the assignments. This guidance may range from facilitating recall of vignettes from participants' experiences that illuminate an aspect of the preceding session to designing rehearsals of new '*in-vivo*' scenarios, in which the assignment requires the implementation of behavioural experiments. They record fully the events of these assignment meetings and pass them on to the practitioners, together with session notes. They act as catalysts for the emergence of new material, help in all group tasks and exercises and operate as memory aids through the notes they take of all proceedings.

- **Group Participants**[2] tend to have an average age of 40 with a range of ±10 years. Their injuries occur between 3 and 10 years prior to joining the programme and include strokes, hypoxias, inflammation of the blood vessels of the brain, haemorrhages and TBIs. Injury severity ranges from moderate to serious, with loss of consciousness lasting from over 40 minutes to a few days, and a post-traumatic amnesia duration of up to and over 3 weeks.

By the time of joining this programme, however, clients have all been discharged from post-acute in-patient rehabilitation lasting up to and over 18 months and are maintained in the community, living either with their families or in assisted living facilities.

All participants are educated at least to GCSE standard. They all have held job roles prior to sustaining their injury ranging across a wide spectrum, including landscape gardening, joinery, teaching, middle management and company directorships.

1.2 Goals, objectives and key concepts

The programme's overarching goal is to retrieve the person behind the injury by helping acquired brain injury survivors master the adverse consequences of their brain injury. It has three key objectives:

- Develop active acceptance and acknowledgment of post-ABI changes
- Rebuild belief in self-efficacy through the experience of goal attainment and of influence and control over events that affect day-to-day life
- Enable generalisation of self-efficacy to situations in which performance was debilitated in consequence of post-ABI change

Two concepts underpin the programme: Frame-breaking change and retrieving the person behind the injury.

- **Frame-breaking change:** This is a concept imported from organisational psychology/ culture change.[3] It is a fitting description of what happens after brain injury. Frame-breaking change impacts the entire system; it causes it to break out of the current pattern of congruence and moves it into a completely new configuration. It is very different from 'frame-bending' or incremental change which impacts parts or components of the system and whose remedial goal is to maintain or to regain pre-change congruence. Incremental change is akin to a broken leg or arm. In that paradigm, it is possible to preserve previous ways of functioning although one's limbs are in plaster. In contrast, in the frame-breaking paradigm of brain injury, the fundamental structure of existing life patterns is destroyed in a way that makes the maintenance of the previous life order impossible. Survivors and families have to learn to live and to adapt to a completely new world configuration.

- **Retrieving the 'person behind the injury':** The primary consequence of the cognitive, emotional and behavioural changes that traumatic brain injury visits upon survivors is to create a watershed that submerges or masks the individual's pre-injury personality. It is as if the person's pre-injury identity that was known to him/her and to family and friends and in social and occupational contexts has fragmented or been annihilated. Depression, anxiety, boredom, loneliness, anomie and alienation characterise the existence of the great majority of survivors grappling with the frame-breaking changes of ABI. Retrieving the person behind the injury in this context refers to rebuilding recognition of and continuity with the pre-ABI self through developing personal autonomy, effectiveness in goal attainment and control over one's life, even as one learns to acknowledge and to accept post-ABI adverse changes.

1.3 Theoretical framework

Cognitive behaviour therapy principles and practice inform this rehabilitation programme. Its working constructs are in two groups: The first group develops awareness and identification of mental events, and the second comprises techniques that achieve behaviour change.

Constructs of self-awareness and identification include core beliefs, assumptions, life rules, protective behaviours and the *metacognitive* concept of the self-regulatory executive.[4] My application of this concept borrows from Jeffrey Young's work[5] on schema therapy. I have used Young's metaphor of conversing with oneself to develop in group participants the ability to stand back and to appraise the parameters of the demand situation and of their own capabilities in relation to it. I have called this conversational partner the Watching Self.

However, rather than examining childhood experiences as the originators of core beliefs, I focus upon the brain injury as the agent that has changed and reshaped systems of pre-existing core belief. Group members explore the ways in which brain injury consequences have transformed their beliefs, assumptions and life rules.

Behaviour change constructs are techniques that include anxiety management, problem-solving strategies and behavioural experiments. Their purpose is to help participants replace dysfunctional coping mechanisms with adaptive ones that will increase the effectiveness with which they adjust to the post-injury order of their life.

The programme's framework is strongly influenced by recent advances in ABI remediation[6] and makes use of concepts such as scaffolding, context sensitivity, metacognition, action learning, generalisation, awareness, locus of control and self-efficacy.[7]

This integrated framework overcomes the fragmentation associated with adherence to stand-alone intervention models and is consistent with the holistic, person-centered priorities of effective rehabilitation.

2 Processes and features

2.1 Selection and progress evaluation

Attendance at these groups is on an outpatient basis, and the culture of community-based facilities tends to favour structured one-on-one clinical discussions over measurement-based selection and progress evaluations.

Initial suitability discussions include taking a personal/medical history and the history of the brain injury, assessing mood-state, reviewing in detail the lifestyles and activities in the here and now, obtaining a profile of strengths and weaknesses, observing interactive skills and examining the ability to generate and to sustain motivation to participate in the programme.

This resource includes a Likert-type rating scale that can be applied at the end of each session. This evaluation lends itself to a cumulative record of progress across the duration of the programme. More importantly, however, the sessions draw examples of participant reports from previous groups. These attest to gains that accrue as the programme develops. Reports of results of behavioural experiments, for example, indicate improved engagement in the various contexts of life leading to increased life quality as the sessions advance. They include:

- **Family-related activities**
  - Improving family relationships
  - Doing the family shopping
  - Helping with/managing the children
  - Preparing/contributing to the preparation of the family meal

- **Work-related activities**
  - Enrolling in voluntary work
  - Attending official meetings
  - Making presentations in meetings

- **Community-related activities**
  - Attending football matches
  - Attending concerts
  - Attending classes
  - Weekends away with friends
  - Negotiating with authorities
  - Making appointments with various health professionals
  - Helping neighbours with tasks

Such narratives have perhaps a stronger evidence base than do rating-scale endorsements.

2.2 Session characteristics

The programme sessions have a standard six-part structure.[8] Part 1 welcomes participants and introduces this session's objectives. Part 2 summarises the previous session and appraises last week's assignment. Part 3 presents that week's topic and engages participants in exercises that spring from it. These exercises facilitate learning and function as practice runs for the following week's assignment.

Parts 4 and 5 are plenaries that review outcomes of exercises and discussions. Part 6 introduces and explains next week's assignment and concludes the session by drawing together its separate strands.

Ground rules are introduced in the first session of the programme titled *Welcome to the Programme*. Within the frame of these rules, sessions are never didactic. They encourage humour and give participants every opportunity to express their views, thoughts and feelings; to communicate their experiences and their doubts; and to share their exercise and assignment results. This practice of disclosure helps participants discover that they are not alone or unique in grappling with the frame-breaking changes of their brain injury. It also develops positive regard and a sense of 'belonging' with each other and with the group.

Session duration is 2 hours on average, but assignment sessions are shorter. There is provision for a 10-minute break halfway through, but no participants in any of my groups have taken this except for brief convenience interludes.[9] Participant numbers vary between five and eight, and two support workers also take part and may act as co-therapists.

3 Resources

3.1 Assignments
The programme is assignment-based and participants are required to complete homework during the one-week interval between sessions. A central task of assignments is to build a bridge between day-to-day life and the content of group sessions. They are especially designed to accomplish this task by facilitating consolidation of learning, motivating participants to apply learned material in real life and report outcome, and developing continuity and relatedness between sessions, and between sessions and the events of the week.

3.2 Session log-files
Participants maintain a session log-file in which they keep programme handouts, session notes and exercises, records of assignments and notes from assignment sessions. Session logs are the depository of the group's continuity and of the individual participant's history within it. Participants are frequently encouraged to refer to their logs and to locate a record of an event within them.

3.3 Programme documents
Each programme session has three companion documents which act as anchors to the modules.[10] These are:

- **Practitioners' Guide** familiarises practitioners with the session aims, tasks and content. It steers them through the session and gives a flavour of likely group atmosphere by acquainting them with participant statements and assignment results from previous groups.
- **Participants' Handout** orients participants to the session. It sets out session objectives, outlines the key activities in each part, introduces and explains that week's topic, presents the session's exercise, gives participants the opportunity to take notes of session events and sets out that week's assignment. Participants complete their assignment with the help of support workers during their assignment session.
- **Support Workers' Guide** steers support workers through the assignment session. It gives cues and clues on facilitating recall of key session events, offers pointers on how to run a discussion about the session and guides them on helping participants complete assignments and evaluations.
- **Evaluation Scale:** Appendix 1 contains this scale for participants to use at the close of each session.

3.4 Other resources
1 Meeting room with table and chairs and sufficient space for group relaxation exercises of Module 3
2 Three flip charts with coloured pens; paper, pencils, biros on table

3 Participants' arch-level files
4 Coffee-/tea-making facilities and conveniences nearby
5 Voice recorder [for Module 3]
6 An appendix at the end of this book contains the evaluation scale for this resource

Notes

1 Taking part in these group sessions will also act as a good training ground for support workers.
2 These are the characteristics of previous groups who have taken part in this programme. They appear to be similar to those attending the Oliver Zangwill Centre (Wilson et al. 2009)
3 Kilmann et al. (1988)
4 Wells (2002) and Teasdale et al. (2002).
5 Young et al. (2003)
6 Cicerone and Azulay (2002), Ylvisaker et al. (2006), Bandura (1977)
7 Ideally, this programme should be delivered as part of an integrated transdisciplinary top-down rehabilitation strategy incorporating cognitive retraining, functional effectiveness retraining and mobility retraining. This was not the case in this instance.
8 But there are exceptions.
9 No participant has ever dropped out of my programme. It is possible, however, to split the sessions if desired; I have never found the need to do so.
10 Except for the first welcome session that has only documents 2 and 3.

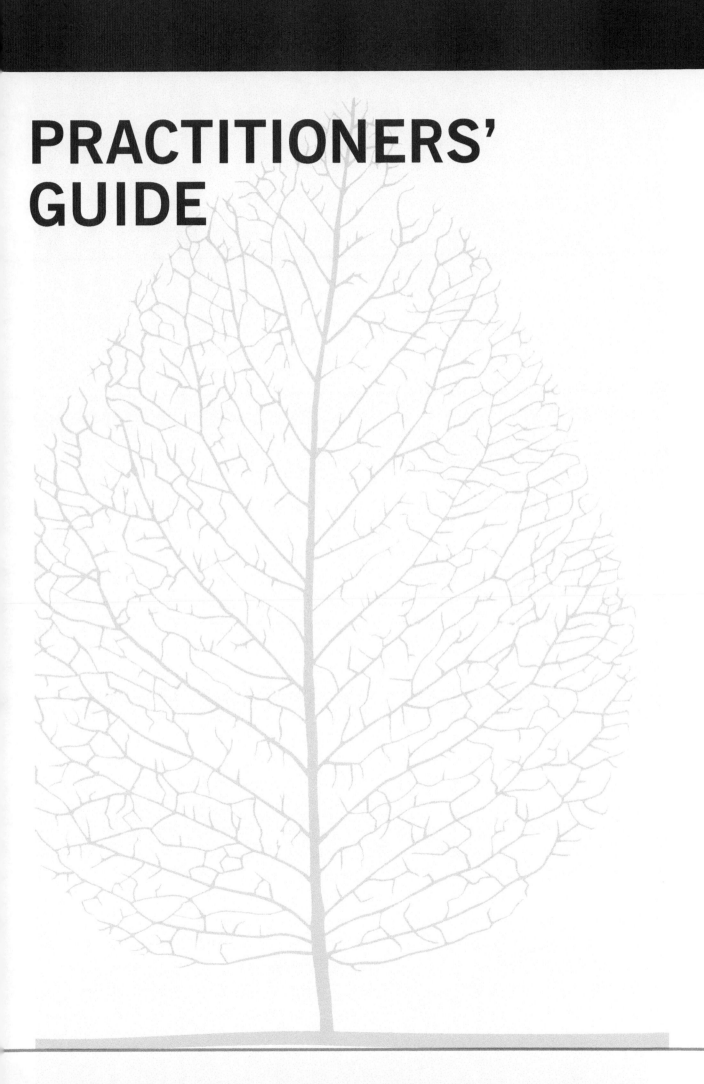

PRACTITIONERS' GUIDE

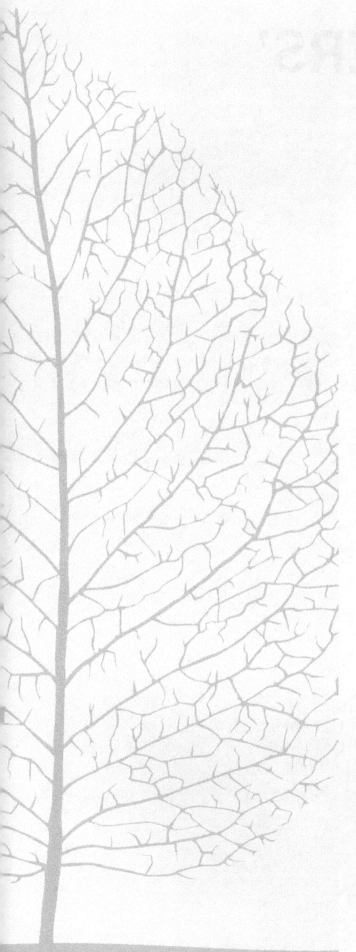

MODULE 1

Recognising change

Practitioners' introduction to module 1

The purpose of this module is to raise participants' awareness of the changes that brain injury has visited upon them. We know that these changes impair functional effectiveness and alter the way people perceive themselves and are perceived by others. Family, social and work relationships deteriorate, and sometimes socio-economic circumstances worsen as well.

Cognitive and emotional impairments together with loss of continuity in the way one experiences oneself create a mindset of helplessness. One of the protective mechanisms which this mindset gives rise to is the 'let sleeping dogs lie' paradigm. This paradigm governs survivors' day-to-day existence and by so doing shields them from moment-to-moment awareness of the devastating impact of their injury upon their sense of selfhood. The cost, however, is that it prevents the mobilisation of adaptive capability because it thwarts recognition, definition and mastery of the frame-breaking changes that occur in post-injury life.

This module's central task is to prepare participants to let go of this paradigm and to lay claim to their lives. The preparation proceeds gently in three stages. First, it helps participants become aware of the pre- and post-injury changes that have taken place in their preference systems; second, it encourages them to think through and to explain why and how these changes have come about. Finally, it urges them to identify which, if any, of these changes create obstacles to the achievement of quality in their lives.

I have used the Myers-Briggs Type Indicator[1] as a tool that facilitates the recognition and definition of change. This is a self-report questionnaire constructed for normal populations. It profiles four psychological preference dimensions relating to how people make relationships, gather information, make decisions and organise their lives. Its basic assumption is that we all have specific preferences in the way we construe our experiences, and these preferences underlie our interests, needs, values and motivation.

The MBTI was developed by Isabel Briggs-Myers and Katherine Briggs in the early 1940s when they both became interested in Carl Jung's type theory.[2]

However, research[3] indicates that the MBTI exhibits significant psychometric deficiencies.

These include poor validity and poor reliability, lack of independence between the four preference dimensions resulting from high intercorrelations, and fairly large standard errors of measurement leading to people being allocated to different preference dimensions despite close proximity of scores.

In this module, I have administered four shortened versions of the MBTI for convenience and ease of understanding. These four questionnaires profile the four preference dimensions individually.

Participant numbers in any one group are small, and the four shortened questionnaires are not standardised. Participants' ratings show prominent pre- and post-ABI differences, but these may fall short of statistical significance and do not follow a consistent pattern. Some preference pairs reverse direction post-ABI and some display substantial intensity changes, either increasing or decreasing.

I do not consider that these shortcomings detract the overarching purpose of this module, namely, to raise participant awareness of change. The function of the MBTI here is solely as a vehicle that articulates the experience of post-ABI difference by making it explicit, intelligible and meaningful.

The module contains five sessions. Session 1 introduces participants to the program. Each of the four sessions beginning with Session 2 focuses on one preference dimension and is in six parts.[4] In Parts 1 and 2, the practitioner welcomes the group and introduces the goals of the session. Part 3 introduces the particular preference dimension and familiarises participants with its polarity by running a 15-minute exercise in which they complete a mini-questionnaire of about eight items. A group discussion of the exercise results follows.

In Part 4, participants complete a questionnaire of between 14 and 18 items and share their results with the group. This is the same questionnaire that they must complete as part of that session's assignment.

Part 5 concentrates on facilitating an in-depth exploration of participants' reasons for post-ABI preference differences. This section gently initiates relevant cognitive behaviour therapy techniques to address the explanations that participants give for change. These include delineation of protective behaviours, rational enquiry, guided exploration and behavioural experiments.

This section also reveals the adverse consequences that may have affected participants' cognitive, affective, motivational and behavioural economies. These include impairments of impulse control, initiation, motivation, working memory, organisation and planning. These consequences may be below the threshold of participants' awareness, and it is beyond the scope of this programme to handle them in detail. However, practitioners must be alert and deal with these issues as they arise outside of this programme.

Finally, Part 6 explains next week's assignment and closes the session by bringing together its various strands

Session 3 and beyond have one additional section that follows Part 2 and facilitates a group summary and review of the previous session and its assignment.

The evaluation scale in the Appendix can be used to rate each session.

Welcome and introduction

➤ AIMS AND OVERVIEW

The central aims of this first session are to draw forth participants' committed engagement to the programme and to plant the seeds of enduring group cohesion. It conveys that this therapeutic enterprise is a safe journey of shared self-discovery.

➤ PROCESS NOTES

Objectives and tasks

Objectives:

1 Encourage commitment by enlisting participant 'buy-in'
2 Plant the seeds of group unity by facilitating exchange of ideas, views and feelings
3 Instil hope that positive outcome can be achieved by reinforcing success narratives

Tasks:

1 Welcome participants, deal with administrative issues and introduce everybody to each other [25 minutes]
2 Introduce the programme [15 minutes]
3 Explore and discuss participant expectations of the programme [20 minutes]
4 Explore and allay participant anxieties about the programme [20 minutes]
5 Set programme ground rules [20 minutes]
6 Encourage participant feedback and close the session [20 minutes]

Total time: 120 minutes

1 Greetings and welcome [25 minutes]

- **Warm welcome**
  - Reference to practitioner-participant one-on-one meeting pre-start as a warm-up

- **Administration**
  - Lever arch files
    - ◆ Description of purpose and use as session logs
    - ◆ Participant preferences for where to keep them[5]
    - ◆ Programme handouts
      - ✧ Description and purpose
      - ✧ Storage in appropriate divider in lever arch file

- **Session outline**
  - Introducing ourselves
  - Overview of programme
  - Expectations and anxieties
  - Ground rules

- **Getting to know each other**
  - My name
  - My brain injury: how, when
  - My life: what was it like before my injury; what was it like immediately post injury; what is it like now

  Participants introduce themselves and receive help with cues and clues as necessary. Support workers take notes of the session. It is important to record participants' self-introduction for later use in the programme.

2 Programme overview [15 minutes]

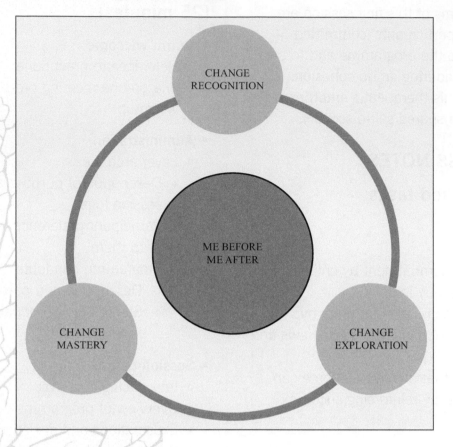

This programme is about recognising, identifying and mastering the changes that the experience of brain injury has brought into our lives. [**Reference to some of the changes that participants gave in their introductions**]. Look at the Overview diagram in your handouts. The 'me before, me after' circle in the centre represents you, and you are what the programme is about. The three circles radiating from it are the programme's modules.

Module 1 deals with helping us to recognise the changes that we have experienced in ourselves as a result of our brain injury. These changes focus on our style of

1 *Making relationships:* **Extrovert/Introvert** [**Extrovert** = being outgoing; having many friends; being the 'life and soul of the party'; wanting to bounce off thoughts and ideas on others to get their views. **Introvert** = having few but good friends; preferring the company of a few people to going to parties and social gatherings; coming to conclusions through reading or talking them through with a few intimate people rather than through discussion/conversation]

2 *Seeking and gathering information:* **Sensing/Intuition** [**Sensing** = getting factual, practical information based on the evidence of our five senses. **Intuition** = going beyond the available practical information and listening to what our 'gut feel' says about things]

3 *Making decisions:* **Thinking/Feeling** [**Thinking** = going over the alternatives carefully one-by-one and arriving at a decision based on logic. **Feeling** = feeling our way through options and deciding which 'feels' right for us]

4 *Organising our lives: our lifestyle:* **Judging/Perceiving** [**Judging** = being well organised; planning things well in advance; being tidy and knowing where everything is; being structured and not leaving anything to chance. **Perceiving** = being easy, laid-back, flexible and spontaneous about things; not planning anything in advance; being slightly untidy; leaving things to the last minute]

In module 2, we explore how and why we have changed since the experience of our brain injury and what the consequences of these changes mean for us. Are we happy about them or do they create obstacles to us getting what we want out of life?

In module 3, we work on learning techniques to master the changes that prevent us from making active choices on how to live our lives.

4 Discussion: participant expectations and anxieties [20 minutes]

- ○ **Expectations**
  - ◆ Is the programme in line with expectations?
  - ◆ Can differences be bridged/aligned? How?
  - ◆ Any other expectations?
  - ◆ Examples of expectations from other groups. Similarities and differences between them and those of this group

- ○ **Anxieties**
  - ◆ Any anxieties?
  - ◆ Examples of anxieties from other groups
  - ◆ Similarities and differences between anxieties of this group and those of others
  - ◆ Can we allay/deal with these anxieties?

5 House rules [20 minutes]

i Commitment

This is your programme. Commit to it. Participate in the group process to the fullest of your ability – personal growth depends on the inclusion of every individual voice. Come on time: do not keep others waiting. Come every week. Call [the clinic] if you cannot make it.

ii Respect

Listen actively – respect others when they are talking. Do ask questions of one another respectfully, but refrain from personal attacks. The goal is not to agree – it is to gain a deeper understanding of ourselves and of each other. Do not invalidate somebody else's story with your own; instead, share your own story and experience with them. Be aware of body language and nonverbal responses – they can be as disrespectful as words. Be supportive of each other. Avoid criticism. Give constructive feedback.

Gossip and secret grudges can be very destructive in a group. If a member has something to say to another group member, they must say it to the member directly rather than talk about him/her behind his/her back. No group member is to be humiliated, undermined or abused in any way. Violence and intimidation towards others are absolutely not allowed.

iii Alcohol and other drugs

Group members cannot participate in the group under the influence of alcohol or other mind-altering drugs. When under the influence of chemicals, persons do not have access to their emotions and have less control over their behaviour. If you appear to be under the influence of alcohol or other drugs, you will be asked to leave the group.

iv Exclusive relationships

Dating and other exclusive relationships between or among group members are not allowed. These relationships split the group and can make other group members feel left out.

v Attendance

You must attend every meeting unless an emergency arises. If an emergency should arise, you should notify [the clinic] to say that you will be unable to attend. If you have three unexcused absences, the group will review your continued group membership.

Sometimes it is necessary for a group member to leave the group unexpectedly. This can cause group members to wonder if they have harmed the leaving member. If you must leave the group unexpectedly, you must come to a last group meeting and tell the members that you are leaving and say goodbye.

You must announce this at the beginning of the last meeting so that the group has time to ask questions and say goodbye. Group members may express their concerns but will respect your decision to leave.

vi Confidentiality

Anything said between any two or more group members at any time is part of the group and is confidential. The names of other members of the group and what is said in the group is confidential to the group. Anything which occurs between or among group members is confidential to the group.

The single exception to this rule of confidentiality applies to the group leader. If the group leader believes that someone is in danger, the leader has a professional obligation to take direct action in order to keep everyone safe.

Anything which occurs between or among any members is part of the group and is not kept secret from the group. It is, however, kept secret from anyone outside of the group. This also applies to any individual meetings you may have with the group leader.

Violating the rule of confidentiality may lead to removal from the group.

vii Assignments

This is an assignment-based programme. Assignments help you to practise what you learn, to increase your self-awareness, and to control your emotions and your behaviours. Almost all sessions will end by asking you to complete assignments, and the session that follows them will begin with an assignment review. You must complete all your assignments. Our support workers will help and support you in this task.

viii Tell me if you are unhappy

Bring your concerns to the group. It is your group, your safe environment. I can't help you if I don't know! Together we can work things out.

6 Discussion of rules, feedback and end [20 minutes]

- **Discussion of rules**
  - Participants' views
  - Any other rules participants wish to propose?

- **Feedback on this session**
- **End**
  - Date time and venue of next session
  - Goodbye

How do I make relationships? extroversion vs. introversion

➤ AIMS AND OVERVIEW

The aim of the second session of this module is to raise participants' awareness of any differences that exist in the way they made relationships before and make them after their acquired brain injury.[6] The session does this by investigating their pre- and post-ABI preference for Extroversion or Introversion.

Extroversion/Introversion is the first of four functions of the Myer-Briggs Type Indicator.[7] It is also the preference which registers the most consistent change after ABI. It is therefore a good beginning to increasing participants' awareness of the changes that have taken place in their self-perceptions pre-and post-ABI.

The Extroversion/Introversion preference is also an exquisite building block of commonality in the group because of the ease with which it elicits shared pre- and post-ABI changes. Group discussion of BEFORE/AFTER ratings is the first step towards participants' self-disclosure and reinforces group cohesion. Participants realise that they are not alone, because their ABI journey is echoed by others in the group. This communicates the universality of the ABI experience, develops a feeling of common history and cultivates a sense of belonging.

The evaluation scale contains a number of questions relating to progress in the activities of daily and community living. In this session, participants are likely to disagree with these. There are not going to be any progress examples given for these activities. Support workers must reassure participants by telling them that it is perfectly acceptable to disagree with some of the statements of the questionnaire.

However, support workers must guard against influencing participant choices and ratings.

➤ PROCESS NOTES

Objectives and tasks

Objectives:

1 Increase participants' awareness of any differences that exist in their pre- and post-ABI preference for Extroversion/ Introversion
2 Help participants put into words the reasons for these differences
3 Identify what, if any, aspects of these differences they wish to change

Tasks:

1 Welcome participants and set out purpose and outline [15 minutes]
2 Introduce the preferences of Extroversion and Introversion [15 minutes]
3 Run a discussion that consolidates understanding of task 2 [20 minutes]
4 Help participants complete the questionnaire, score their ratings and record them on a flip chart [15 minutes]
5 Give feedback and lead a discussion on:
   Is how I make relationships now different from how I made them before my brain injury? [30 minutes]
6 Set next week's assignment and end the session [15 minutes]

Total time: 110 minutes

How do I make relationships? extroversion vs. introversion

1 Welcome and introduction [15 minutes]

- Introduce session and check session logs are in order
- Distribute and explain session handouts with help from support workers
- State session objectives and outline
- Briefly discuss and get agreement on session structure

2 Extroversion and introversion [15 minutes]

Extroversion and Introversion are a pair of psychological preferences. They relate primarily to relationship making. Extroverts get their energy from the outside world, the world of people and things. Introverts get their energy from the inner world, the world of ideas and images.

Extrovert people are sociable, outgoing and have many friends. They take the initiative in making new friends; they like meeting new people and can be the life and soul of the party. They like to be involved in many groups and activities, welcome change, make quick decisions and don't like to be alone.

Introvert people are deep thinkers, who have to consider the ins and outs of situations before they make decisions. They have few but close friends. They tend to prefer to be alone and involve themselves in solitary activities. They prefer to read rather than to meet people. They do not like change and can work alone for long periods.

3 Discussion: me before – me after [20 minutes; handout page 5]

- **Where did you get your main source of energy BEFORE ABI? Where do you get your main source of energy AFTER ABI?** Was it/is it the world outside you, the world of people and things, or your inner world, the world of ideas and images?
- **Look at the graphic on page 12 of your handouts: Which figure has a strong extrovert preference; which figure has a strong introvert preference? Which one is most like you before ABI? Which one is most like you after ABI?** Facilitated group description of the graphic. [Both figures are full of ideas, but ideas are bursting out of the head and mouth of the figure on the left. Ideas are deep within the head of the figure on the right.]

4 Completing the questionnaire and feedback [15 minutes]

- **Explanation of instructions**
- **Flip-chart table**
- **Result read-out and recording**
- **Feedback discussion:**
  - **Example from previous groups:**
    Most survivors rate themselves as having been extrovert pre-ABI and having become introvert after it. The reasons they give for having changed include loss of confidence, loss of purpose, loss of drive and worrying about what people think.
    Table 1 offers an example of participant exercise ratings.

How do I make relationships? extroversion vs. introversion

Table 1 Example of participant ratings on the preference of Extrovert/Introvert

Participant[8]	Score After ABI		Score Before ABI	
	Extrovert	Introvert	Extrovert	Introvert
1	3	8	8	3
2	4	7	7	4
3	5	6	9	2
4	2	9	8	3
5	5	6	7	4

○ **Discussion topics:**
  ♦ Exploring reasons for change
  ♦ Did you have similar concerns pre-ABI?
  ♦ If not, why do you have them now?
  ♦ If you had similar concerns pre-ABI, were they as intense as they are now, post-ABI?

5 Next week's assignment and end [15 minutes]

Assignment 1: EXTROVERT/INTROVERT: Please complete this questionnaire by putting a cross beside the item that describes you best for both **AFTER** and **BEFORE** your ABI. Please answer every question. When you finish, add up your crosses in each column. Work out also the grand total of your crosses and put them in the appropriate columns at the end of the continuation table.

Assignment 2: HOW HAVE I CHANGED? Please summarise the ways in which you have changed in your own words: the way you see yourself now, after your brain injury, compared with the way you saw yourself then, before your brain injury. I have given three examples to get you started.

Assignment 3: Based on Tables 1 and 2, please identify and list the changes you want to make about yourself after your ABI.

This session does not broach Assignment 3 [page 10 of handout]. This is the task in which participants identify and list the BEFORE/AFTER changes in their Extroversion/Introversion preferences that they would like to remedy. The purpose of this unrehearsed task is to encourage participants early in the programme to take the initiative in thinking about the future and about the goals they wish to achieve.

How do I make relationships? extroversion vs. introversion

EXERCISE

EXTROVERT/INTROVERT: Please complete this questionnaire by putting a cross beside the item that describes you best for both **AFTER** and **BEFORE** your ABI. Please answer every question. When you finish, add up your crosses in each column. Work out also the grand total of your crosses and put them in the appropriate columns at the end of the continuation table.

Table 2

Extroversion [E]	After ABI X	Before ABI X	Introversion [I]	After ABI X	Before ABI X
1 I like getting my energy from taking active part in what is going on around me			1 I like getting my energy from dealing with what is inside my own head: my own ideas, memories, images and reactions that are in my inner world		
2 I like it when there are lots of people around me			2 I often prefer doing things alone or with one or two people I feel comfortable with		
3 I like taking action and making things happen			3 I take time to think things through so that I have a clear idea of what I'll be doing when I decide to act		
4 I generally feel part of the world around me and feel at home in it			4 I feel most comfortable and 'at home' in my own company or in the company of one or two people that I know well		
5 I often understand a problem better when I can talk out loud about it and hear what others have to say			5 I feel comfortable solving my problems on my own		
6 I am a 'people person'			6 I am 'reserved' and tend to keep myself to myself		
TOTAL					

(Continued)

How do I make relationships? extroversion vs. introversion

Table 2 (Continued)

	After ABI	Before ABI		After ABI	Before ABI
Extroversion [E]	X	X	**Introversion [I]**	X	X
7 I feel comfortable in groups of people and like doing things in them			**7** I feel comfortable being alone and like things I can do on my own		
8 I have a wide range of friends and know lots of people			**8** I prefer to know just a few people well		
9 I sometimes jump too quickly into an activity and don't allow enough time to think it over			**9** I sometimes spend too much time thinking things through and don't move into action quickly enough		
10 Before I start a project, I sometimes forget to stop and get clear on what I want to do and why			**10** I sometimes forget to check with the outside world to see if my ideas really fit the experience		
11 I would change the world if I could			**11** I would understand the world if I could		
TOTAL					
GRAND TOTAL					

How do I gather information? sensing vs. intuition

➤ AIMS AND OVERVIEW

The aim of this third session is to increase participants' awareness of any differences that exist in the way they gather information before and after their acquired brain injury by profiling their pre- and post-ABI preferences for Sensing and Intuition.

The Sensing and Intuition scale of the MBTI presents difficulties.[9] Research[10] indicates that only the Extroversion and Introversion scale has strong validity because it shows high correlations with other instruments that assess comparable personality dimensions but low correlations with those that profile different personality dimensions. In contrast, the statistical properties of the Sensing and Intuition scale are weak. It is therefore important for practitioners to ensure that this scale is effective in raising awareness of BEFORE/AFTER changes by helping participants to understand fully the concepts it purports to measure.

Day-to-day information gathering happens so quickly that people hardly register the activity even whilst engaging in it. Most people tend to overlook its significance in decision-making. This session spends some time on exploring this activity in concrete terms to enable the group to develop a clear understanding of the dichotomous preferences associated with it.

Participants generally rate the **AFTER ABI** direction of their Sensing/Intuition preferences as having stayed the same but the intensity as having changed.

Whilst modules 2 and 3 of the programme will deal with the feasibility aspect of participants' reasons for post-ABI change,

this session gently begins to introduce the techniques of rational enquiry and guided discovery. For example, how realistic is it for participants to rely on intuition alone, because of impaired eyesight/memory? Is it realistic to expect absolute safety or to expect never to do anything wrong?

➤ PROCESS NOTES

Objectives and tasks

Objectives:

1 Identify Pre- and post-ABI preference differences in information gathering
2 Help put into words the reasons for these differences
3 Help identify what, if any, aspects of these differences they wish to change

Tasks:

1 Welcome participants, set out the purpose and outline of the session [10 minutes]
2 Summarise last week's session and review assignments [20 minutes]
3 Draw attention to the importance of information gathering and introduce the preferences of Sensing and Intuition [40 minutes]
4 **'Which type are you?'** Help participants complete and score their questionnaire ratings and record ratings on flip chart [15 minutes]
5 Give feedback and lead a discussion on: **Is how I gather information now different from how I did before my brain injury?** [30 minutes]
6 Set next week's assignment and end this session [10 minutes]

Total time: 125 minutes

How do I gather information?
sensing vs. intuition

1 Welcome and introduction [10 minutes]

As set out in task list

2 Summary of last session and assignment review [20 minutes]

- **Last session**
  - Recall and discussion of key points of last session
  - Discussion on how participants' experiences of the week confirm or otherwise this material

- **Assignment review**
  - **Examples from previous groups** tend to confirm participants' within-session self-ratings for Extroversion/Introversion. In my groups of between six and eight participants, 71 percent dropped their **BEFORE ABI** Extroversion scores by between three and eight points and increased their **AFTER ABI** Introversion scores by between one and seven points. Tables 3 and 4 offer typical assignment ratings and change goals.

Table 3 BEFORE/AFTER group scores

| | Before | | After | | Before | After |
	Extrovert	Introvert	Extrovert	Introvert	Preference Change	Preference Change
1	6	7	3 −3	6 −1	I	I
2	7	0	6 −1	6 +6	E	=
3	6	3	2 −4	5 +2	E	I
4	8	4	5 −3	6 +2	E	I
5	8	6	6 −2	3 −3	E	E
6	8	3	3 −5	10 +7	E	I
7	4	0	6 +2	6 +6	E	I

Table 4 Example of participant goals

Participant	Goals
1	• Improve walking, talking, balance and initiative
2	• Stop keeping feelings to myself • Say what I feel
3	• Improve motivation • Explore possibilities for voluntary work
4	• Stop being stubborn • Relax more • Stop trying to always organise things • Stop getting anxious

(Continued)

How do I gather information? sensing vs. intuition

Table 4 (Continued)

Participant	Goals
5	• Stop worrying about what others think • Stop worrying about being late • Increase motivation • Control temper
6	• Go out more • Stop worrying about crowds • Stop worrying about what others think

- **Present group**
    - Tables 1 and 2: Participants read out their BEFORE/AFTER assignment ratings. Group discussion on whether these are different from last week's within-session ratings. If yes, why? If not, how do they explain the consistent BEFORE/AFTER differences? How do these relate to their ratings on Assignment Table 2?
    - Table 3: Participants read out what they would like to change about their BEFORE/ AFTER differences from Table 3
    - Participants link assignment review results to their experiences during the week

3 How we gather information: sensing and intuition [40 minutes]
- **Description**

    Sensing and intuition are information-gathering functions. They describe how we collect, understand and process information. Give me some examples of what information you have sought and gathered during the past week.

    - ♦ **Mini Discussion [05 minutes]**

        Participants give examples of what information they have gathered during the week [studying bus timetable, checking diary, reading recipe].

People who prefer sensing, trust information that is in the present, tangible and concrete; that is, information that can be understood by the five senses. They tend to distrust hunches which seem to come 'out of nowhere.' They prefer to look for details and facts. For them, the meaning is in the here and now and in the facts. They pay attention to physical reality, what they see, hear, touch, taste and smell. They are concerned with what is actual, present, current and real. They are good with their hands, and like to get on with the task at hand. They are not interested in what might happen in the future or what might be possible. They do not think of **what might happen tomorrow or next week if . . .** They look at **what is actually happening now**.

People who prefer intuition, on the other hand, trust information that is less dependent upon the senses. They pay attention to impressions or to the meaning and patterns of the information they get. They prefer to learn by thinking a problem through than by hands-on experience. They are interested in new things and what might be possible. They remember events more as an impression of what it was like than as actual facts or details of what happened.

How do I gather information? sensing vs. intuition

They concentrate on the future and on possibilities. They are always thinking **what might happen if . . .** They are less interested in what is going on in the here and now. They are imaginative and have many 'gut feels.'

When they solve a problem, they look at many more options than might be necessary because they want to be sure that they have not missed anything that **might be relevant in the future or might go wrong in the future.**

For example, if a sensing person is buying a house, he/she gets on with it without looking at the future plans for the area. A sensing type will simply concern herself with the dimensions and properties of the house in the here and now. She will not concern herself with whether the house will lose or gain in value in 10 years' time because of changes in the locality.

An intuitive person, on the other hand, will look at all the future options before making the decision to buy. He or she will remember her previous houses and how she hoped to furnish her next house. She will be more interested in what might happen to the house in 10 years' time.

Both types have their advantages and disadvantages. An intuitive person may never get to buy the house because he/she will take so long gathering the information that it may be sold to another buyer. A sensing person may buy it quickly and find that in 10 years' time a motorway will be built and the house will be demolished.

4 Exercise: which type are you? [15 minutes]

• **Completing the questionnaire**

Do you pay more attention to information that comes in through your five senses **(Sensing)**, or do you pay more attention to the patterns and possibilities that you see in the information you receive **(Intuition)**? Put a cross on the statement that applies to you best. Participants rate their preferences as they are now, AFTER ABI, and read out their results. These are noted on a flip chart as below.

	Sensing [S]	Intuition [N]
1		
2		
3		
4		
5		
6		
7		

After this mini-practice trial participants complete the questionnaire.

• **Feedback**

Follow the same procedure as in the previous session.

How do I gather information?
sensing vs. intuition

EXERCISE

SENSING/INTUITION: Please complete this questionnaire by putting a cross beside the item that describes you best for both **AFTER** and **BEFORE** your ABI. Please answer every question. When you finish, add up your crosses in each column. Work out also the grand total of your crosses and put them in the appropriate columns at the end of the continuation table.

Sensing [S]	After ABI	Before ABI	Intuition [N]	After ABI	Before ABI
	X	X		X	X
1 I remember events as a series of photographs of what actually happened			1 I remember events by what I read 'between the lines' about their meaning		
2 I pay attention to physical reality			2 I am interested in doing things that are new and different		
3 I look at the facts to solve a problem			3 I like to see the big picture before I settle down to thinking about the facts		
4 I am a here-and-now person; I just concentrate on what is happening now			4 I trust impressions, symbols, and gut-feel more than what I actually experience through my senses		
5 I start with what is here now; I am not interested in what might happen later			5 I solve problems by thinking through possible solutions rather than by trying them out		
6 I trust experience and actions; I am not interested in words and symbols			6 I am a future-oriented person; not a here-and-now person		
TOTAL					

(Continued)

How do I gather information? sensing vs. intuition

Sensing [S]	Before ABI	After ABI	Intuition [N]	Before ABI	After ABI
	X	X		X	X
7 When I have a problem, I look at the options that are present now; I am not interested in what options may present in the future			7 I concentrate on what might happen rather than on what is		
8 Sometimes I pay so much attention to facts that I miss possibilities			8 I prefer the theoretical to the practical		
9 I value things that are useful			9 I am imaginative and have many gut-feels		
10 I learn best by doing things rather than by reading about them			10 When I solve a problem, I consider many more options than are necessary because I want to make sure that I have not missed anything that might go wrong in the future		
11 When I have a problem, I look at the options that are present now; I am not interested in what options may present in the future			11 I trust my impressions about things rather than my senses		
12 Sometimes I pay so much attention to facts that I miss possibilities			12 I concentrate on what might happen rather than on what is		
13 I make decisions based on what my senses tell me here and now; I do not take any notice of my impressions			13 I value things that are beautiful and meaningful; their usefulness is not important		
TOTAL					
GRAND TOTAL					

How do I gather information? sensing vs. intuition

5 Discussion: is how I gather information now different from how I did before my brain injury? [30 minutes]

- Identification of individual before/after similarities and differences
- Discussion of the reasons for similarities and differences
- Are there any coping mechanisms associated with these similarities and differences? What difficulties do they help you cope with? How do they help you cope with these difficulties?

6 Next week's assignment and end [10 minutes]

Follow the procedure of the last session.

How do I make decisions? thinking vs. feeling

➤ AIMS AND OVERVIEW

This session's aim is to increase participants' awareness of any differences that exist in the way they make decisions before and after their acquired brain injury.

Thinking/Feeling preferences register more frequent directional change in my groups than do Sensing/Intuition preferences. However, the direction of post-ABI change is not consistent across participants. Exploring the reasons for change opens a window of understanding on how the group manages its post-ABI problems. For example, would an increased preference for Feeling suggest a similar post-ABI preference increase for Intuition, or the opposite? Could protective mechanisms be at play here? Are the reasons participants give for post-ABI change in decision-making the same as those they gave for information gathering? Is this a sign of adaptive change, or does it suggest well-established protective mechanisms, or could it be an example of perseverative or narrowed thought patterns?

➤ PROCESS NOTES

Objectives and tasks

Objectives:

1 Increase participants' awareness of any differences that exist in the way they make decisions before and after their acquired brain injury
2 Help put into words the reasons for these differences
3 Help identify what, if any, aspects of these differences they wish to change

Tasks:

1 Welcome participants, set out its purpose and outline [10 minutes]
2 Summarise last week's session and review assignments [15 minutes]
3 Describe the preferences of Thinking and Feeling [40 minutes]
4 Help participants complete the questionnaire and record their ratings on a flip chart [15 minutes]
5 Give feedback and facilitate a discussion on: **Is how I make decisions now different from how I made them before my brain injury?** [30 minutes]
6 Explain next week's assignment and end the session [15 minutes]

Total time: 125 minutes

1 Welcome and introduction [10 minutes]

As set out in task list

2 Summary of last session and assignment review [15 minutes]

- **Last session**
  - Recall and discussion of key points of last session
  - Discussion on how participants' experiences of the week confirm or otherwise this material

- **Assignment review**
  - **Examples from previous groups** tend to confirm participants' within-session self-ratings for Sensing and Intuition. Discussion with support workers on assignment sessions also confirms participants' within-session explanations of pre- and post-ABI differences. Tables 5 and 6 set out typical participant ratings and explanations for change.

How do I make decisions?
thinking vs. feeling

Table 5 BEFORE/AFTER Sensing/Intuition ratings of one group

	Before		After		Preference	
	Sensing	Intuition	Sensing	Intuition	Before	After
1	9	9	2	2	=	=
2	6	6	5	5	=	=
3	4	3	7	6	S	S
4	8	8	4	8	=	N
5	6	6	8	5	=	S
6	11	3	8	4	S	S
7	6	6	9	1	=	S

Table 6 Reasons for Sensing/Intuition intensity change AFTER ABI

	Intensity	Within-Session Reason	Assignment Reason
1	Both reduced	Not motivated to gather information; don't care	I don't look at much information before I make a decision; not interested
2	No change		I use both sense and intuition but make fewer decisions because I don't trust myself
3	Both increased	I am more cautious; I require more information for safety	I make many more decisions than pre-ABI because I am more concerned about my safety
4	S reduced	I don't trust my senses; poor eyesight; poor memory; I rely wholly on my intuition	I am more cautious; I get upset if I get things wrong; my senses let me down; I rely more on my feelings
5	S increased	I am more careful; I need information to be sure	I trust my intuition much less because I am less confident
6	S reduced	Not motivated to gather information	I turn a blind eye and let sleeping dogs lie; I do not take any notice of my intuition
7	S increased	I don't trust intuition; I need more information to avoid mistakes and getting things wrong	I need to look at things more carefully before I do them

- **Present group**
  - ◆ Tables 5 and 6: Participants read out their BEFORE/AFTER assignment ratings. Group discussion on whether these are different from last week's within-session ratings. If yes, why? If not, how do they explain the consistent BEFORE/AFTER differences? How do these relate to their ratings on Assignment Table 6?
  - ◆ For example, the need for more information may reflect a protective mechanism related to the negative consequences of ABI; lack of motivation may link to a general loss of initiative which in turn may adversely impact functional effectiveness

- Table 7: Participants read out what they would like to change about their BEFORE/AFTER differences from Table 7
- Participants link assignment review results to their experiences during the week

3 How we make decisions: thinking and feeling [40 minutes]

- **Description**

A 'Thinker' makes decisions in a rational, logical, impartial manner, based on what they believe to be fair and correct by pre-defined rules of behaviour.

A 'Feeler' makes decisions on the individual case, in a subjective manner, based on what they believe to be right within their own value systems.

For example, say you are a nurse, a doctor, a firefighter. Your organisation imposes a pay cut on you that you think is unjust. Would you go on strike to ensure fair pay, even though you know that the public depends on your services? Or would you carry on working, although you know that this may cause you and some of your colleagues a lower standard of living despite your hard work? **[Facilitated brief discussion of 5 minutes]**

When someone makes a decision that is based on logic and reason, they are operating in **Thinking** mode. When someone makes a decision that is based on their value system, or what they believe to be right, they are operating in **Feeling** mode. We all use both modes for making decisions, but we put more trust into one mode or the other.

Thinking people analyse the given facts and arrive at a decision through a logical thinking process. They tend to make decisions quite quickly and are not interested in how people will be affected by their decisions. They can make quite tough decisions, such as sacking people, for example.

They focus on making the best decision that will be the best solution to the problem at hand. They are not interested in the moral implications of such decisions or if people's feelings will be hurt by the consequences of their decision.

Feeling people are person-oriented and concerned with the moral implications of their decisions. They focus on the feelings of the individuals that will be affected by their decisions. They are concerned that their decisions uphold the principles of justice, fairness and morality. Because of this, feeling-focused people tend to take a long time to make decisions. They want to make sure that their decision does not violate a moral principle in which they have a strong belief.

Decisions that we find most difficult are those in which we **have conflicts** between our **Thinking** and **Feeling** sides. In these situations, our dominant preference will take over. Decisions which we find easy to make and feel good about are usually a result of being in synchrony between our **Feeling** and **Thinking** sides.

4 Exercise: which type are you? [15 minutes]

Follow the same procedure as in the previous session.

How do I make decisions?
thinking vs. feeling

THINKING/FEELING: Please complete this questionnaire by putting a cross beside the item that describes you best for both **AFTER** and **BEFORE** your ABI. Please answer every question. When you finish, add up your crosses in each column. Work out also the grand total of your crosses and put them in the appropriate columns at the end of the continuation table.

Table 7

Thinking [T]	After ABI	Before ABI	Feeling [F]	After ABI	Before ABI
	X	X		X	X
1 I make decisions quite quickly because I am concerned about solving the problem as quickly as possible without spending too much time on how this will impact the people concerned			**1** I take a long time to make decisions because I want to make sure that my decision does not violate any moral principles and upsets the people concerned as little as possible		
2 I make decisions in a rational, logical, impartial manner, based on what I believe to be fair and correct by pre-defined rules of behaviour			**2** I make decisions on the individual case, in a subjective manner based on what I believe to be right within my own value system		
3 I am a solution-oriented person and make decisions by analysing the given facts. I focus on making the best decision that will be the best solution to the problem at hand. I am not interested in the moral implications of such decisions or if people's feelings will be hurt by its consequences.			**3** I am a people-oriented person and take care to make sure that the implications of my decisions do not violate the moral principles in which I believe		
TOTAL					

(Continued)

How do I make decisions? thinking vs. feeling

Table 7 (Continued)

Thinking [T]	After ABI	Before ABI	Feeling [F]	After ABI	Before ABI
	X	X		X	X
4 When I make decisions, I like to rely on facts and impersonal information irrespective of how my decisions might affect the people concerned			4 When I make decisions, I like to think of how it will affect the people concerned and how they are likely to feel		
5 When I make decisions, I like to be impersonal; I do not let my personal wishes or other people's wishes influence me			5 When I make decisions, I take into account what people care about and take account of the viewpoints of the people involved in the situation		
6 I like to make decisions on technical and factual matters where I can use my logic			6 I like to make decisions in matters where it is important to establish what is best for people and where I can rely on the principles of what is right and what is wrong		
7 I believe that telling the truth is more important than being tactful about people's feelings			7 When I make decisions, I like to make sure that I maintain harmony between people		
8 When I make decisions I sometimes ignore or do not value the 'people' aspect of the situation			8 I believe that being tactful about people's feelings is more important than telling the 'cold truth'		
9 I look for logical solutions or explanations to everything			9 I look for what is important to others and express concern for others		

(Continued)

How do I make decisions?
thinking vs. feeling

Table 7 (Continued)

Thinking [T]	After ABI	Before ABI	Feeling [F]	After ABI	Before ABI
	X	X		X	X
10 I make decisions with my head and want to be fair			10 I make decisions with my heart and want to be compassionate		
11 Others sometimes see me as too task-focused and uncaring or indifferent			11 Others sometimes see me as too idealistic, soft or indirect		
TOTAL					
GRAND TOTAL					

5 Discussion: is how I make decisions now after my brain injury different from how I did before my brain injury? [30 minutes]
- **What are pre- and post-ABI changes?**
- **Exploring reasons for change**
  - Are the reasons for change in Thinking/Feeling preferences similar or different from those in Sensing/Intuition?
  - How do these reasons for change compare with those between Extroversion/Introversion?
  - Do these changes represent the way we cope with our post-ABI life demands?

6 Next week's assignment and end [15 minutes]
Follow the procedure of the last session.

How do I organise my life? judging vs. perceiving

➤ AIMS AND OVERVIEW

This is the fifth and last session of Module 1. Its aims are first, to increase participants' awareness of any differences that exist in the way they organise their lives before and after their acquired brain injury, and second, to prepare them for the next module.

The first aim combines participants' post-ABI preferences into a 'lifestyle' and highlights how this differs from their pre-ABI lifestyle. For example, reduced extroversion, information gathering and decision-making would configure into a helpless, withdrawn life that lacks initiative and motivation. The opposite may suggest a rather disinhibited, disorganised mode of living.

The preparation for module 2 points out that now that we have recognised and acknowledged the frame-breaking changes consequent upon our experience with ABI, we are ready to explore how we deal with them in our day-to-day lives.

➤ PROCESS NOTES

Objectives and tasks

Objectives:

1 Increase participants' awareness of any differences that exist in the way they organised their lives before and after their acquired brain injury
2 Help put into words the reasons for these differences
3 Help identify what, if any, aspects of these differences they wish to change

4 Raise participants' awareness that this is the last session of Module 1 and prepare them for Module 2

Tasks:

1 Welcome participants, set out the session's purpose and outline [10 minutes]
2 Summarise last week's session and review assignments [20 minutes]
3 **'How do you organise your life?'** Introduce the preferences of Judging and Perceiving [30 minutes]
4 Help participants complete the questionnaire, score their ratings, and record scores on flip chart [15 minutes]
5 Facilitate a discussion on:
 Is how I organise my life now different from how I did before my brain injury? [30 minutes]
6 Set next week's assignment; explain to participants that this is the last session of this module, introduce the next module and end the session [15 mins]

Total time: 120 minutes

1 Welcome [10 minutes]
As set out in task list

2 Summary of last session and assignment review [20 minutes]
- **Last session**
  - Recall and discussion of key points of last session
  - Discussion on how participants' experiences of the week confirm or otherwise this material
- **Assignment review**
  - **Examples from previous groups:** Table 8 sets out typical pre- and post-ABI preference ratings for Thinking and Feeling

How do I organise my life?
judging vs. perceiving

Table 8 Thinking/Feeling self-rating differences of one group

	Post-ABI			Pre-ABI		
	Thinking	**Feeling**	**Preference**	**Thinking**	**Feeling**	**Preference**
1	9 +7	2 −7	T	2	9	F
2	6 −3	5 +3	T	9	2	T
3	3 −5	8 +5	F	8	3	T
4	8 +3	3 −3	T	5	6	F
5	3 −5	8 +5	F	8	3	T
6	2 −5	9 +5	F	7	4	T

- ○ **Present group**
  - ♦ Table 8: Participants read out their BEFORE/AFTER assignment ratings
  - ♦ Table 9: Participants read out what they would like to change about their BEFORE/AFTER differences
- • **Discussion**
  - ○ Are assignment ratings different from last week's within-session rating? If yes, why? If not, how do they explain the consistent BEFORE/AFTER differences? How do these relate to their ratings on Assignment Table 2?
  - ○ Exploring reasons for change
    - ♦ Do changes in Thinking/Feeling polarities find echo in changes in other preference pairs? What may such changes mean?
    - ♦ Would an increased post-ABI preference for Feeling, for example, suggest a similar post-ABI preference increase for Intuition, or the opposite?
    - ♦ Participants link assignment review results to their experiences during the week

3 How we organise our lives: judging and perceiving [30 minutes]

- • **Description**

  Today we will look at how we organised our lives before we had our brain injury and how we do so now, after our injury. The two preference pairs are **Judging** and **Perceiving**.

  What was your lifestyle before you had your ABI? What is it now? Your lifestyle is what others tend to see about your life. Do others see you as having everything in good order and nicely arranged? Your room is neat and tidy, your desk is clear of papers, your day is structured so that you know at all times what you are meant to do and where you are meant to go.

  Or, do others see you as rather untidy and disorganised? Your desk is full of papers and your room is in a mess. You are late for appointments because something new that has

How do I organise my life?
judging vs. perceiving

come your way sidetracks you. You plan nothing in advance and you enjoy the chaos you are in. **[Facilitated brief discussion of 5 minutes]**

Judging people like to plan everything and do not like the unexpected to be sprung upon them. Their holidays are arranged well in advance, their appointments are set in advance and they are extremely punctual. They are highly organised and highly efficient. They do not like to change their programme or plans to fit in with something new and they certainly do not like last-minute changes.

Perceiving people are rather disorganised although they know where everything is. Their desks are full of papers that require attention and their rooms tend to be in need of putting in order. They do not like to commit to advance plans and consider the unexpected as a welcome challenge. They are easily adaptable and like to learn new ways of doing things. They tend not to keep time or appointments well because they easily attend to something new that has

come their way. They tend not to plan their holidays or anything in advance and thrive on chaos.

Judgers approach life in a structured way, creating plans and organizing their world to achieve their goals and desired results in a predictable way. They like to take charge of their environment and to make choices early. They are self-disciplined and decisive, and like to make decisions quickly and get the job done.

Perceivers look upon structure as being limiting. They prefer to keep their choices open so they can cope with the many problems that life will put in their way. They are curious and like to expand their knowledge. They are tolerant of other people's differences and will adapt to fit into whatever the situation requires. They tend to avoid or put off decisions and instead prefer to explore problems and situations.

4 Exercise: Which type are you? [15 minutes]

Follow the same procedure as in the previous session.

How do I organise my life?
judging vs. perceiving

Table 9 EXERCISE

JUDGING/PERCEIVING: Please put a cross beside the item that describes you best **AFTER** and **BEFORE** your ABI. Please answer every question. When you finish, add up your crosses in each column. Work out also the grand total of your crosses and put them in the appropriate columns at the end of the continuation table.

Judging [J]	After ABI	Before ABI	Perceiving [P]	After ABI	Before ABI
	X	X		X	X
1 I prefer a planned, orderly way of life			1 I prefer a flexible, spontaneous way of life		
2 I like to have things settled and organised			2 I like to understand the world rather than to organise it		
3 I like to bring life under control as much as possible			3 I am always open to new experiences and to new ways of doing things		
4 I like to have things decided			4 I tend to decide what to do as I do it rather than make a plan in advance		
5 I like to know what the task is and get on with it			5 I am loose and casual; I don't like to plan things in advance		
6 I like to make lists of things to do			6 I don't like to separate work and play; I like to mix them		
7 I like to get my work done before playing			7 I work in bursts of energy		
8 I avoid deadlines by planning my work well in advance			8 I am stimulated by an approaching deadline so I never plan my work		
9 Sometimes I focus so much on making the decision that I miss new information			9 I like the unexpected and look upon it as a welcome challenge		

(Continued)

How do I organise my life?
judging vs. perceiving

Table 9 (Continued)

Judging [J]	After ABI	Before ABI	Perceiving [P]	After ABI	Before ABI
	X	X		X	X
10 I don't like unexpected things to be sprung upon me			10 I am not very punctual because I get sidetracked by new things that come my way		
11 I don't like last-minute changes			11 My house is generally in a mess but I like it that way		
12 I make sure my house is always in good order			12 Sometimes I stay open to new information too long, and I miss making important decisions		
13 I schedule things well in advance			13 I postpone making decisions because I want to see what other options are available		
14 I like to make a decision about an issue quickly so that I can move on			14 I like to do things at the last minute		
15 Others see me as well organised but not always flexible			15 Others see me as disorganised but I know where everything is		
16 I am always punctual and structured			16 I don't like to commit to plans too far in advance		
TOTAL					
GRAND TOTAL					

How do I organise my life?
judging vs. perceiving

5 Discussion: is how I organise my life now after my brain injury different from how I did before my brain injury? [30 minutes]

- **What are pre- and post-ABI changes?**
- **Exploring reasons for change**
  - Do you think that the post-ABI increase in your Judging preference helps you to cope better? In what way?
  - What about increases in your Perceiving preference? Does not being so structured help you? How does it do so?
  - How do the reasons for change between Judging/Perceiving compare with those between Thinking/Feeling, Sensing/Intuition and Extroversion/Introversion?
  - Do these changes represent the way we cope with our post-ABI life demands?

6 Next week's assignment and end [15 minutes]

- **Mini-group discussion on this last session of Module 1**
  - Review of areas of post-ABI change
  - Summary of Module 2 activities
    - How and why have we changed since our brain injury?
    - What are the consequences of these changes?
    - Are we happy about these changes or do they present us with obstacles in attaining our life goals?
    - Recapture of Programme Overview Diagram [Session 1, page 6]
- **This week's assignments**
  - **Purpose:**
    - Prepare you for module 2 of the programme
  - **Tasks:**
    - **Assignment 1:**
      - ✧ Complete the questionnaire

- ✧ Add up your scores
- ✧ Are your ratings any different from those of now?
- **Assignment 2:** describe in your own words how and why you have changed.
- **Assignment 3:** go through your session log and record your pre- and post-ABI preferences on all four dimensions together with your pre- and post-ABI ratings.
- **Assignment 4:** record the first letter of each of your four pre- and post-ABI preferences and give a short summary of how you have changed on all four of them.
- **Assignment 5:** Identify the preferences which you wish to change back to the way they were pre-ABI.
  - **Facilitated brief discussion to check participant understanding**

Notes

1 MBTI: Consulting Psychologists Press, Inc. (1998)
2 Jung (1971)
3 Pittenger (2005)
4 Except for Session 2 which is in five parts because it has no assignment section
5 It may be preferable for the facility to keep the files as the participants may lose them or leave them at home.
6 Hereafter referred to as ABI
7 MBTI: It is beyond the scope of this workbook to debate the biologic determinants of the four functions. Looking upon them as preferences that individuals are able to change is the most effective way of achieving the goals of this module.
8 Names have been replaced by numbers.
9 This is also the case with the decision-making and lifestyle scales.
10 Pittenger (2005)

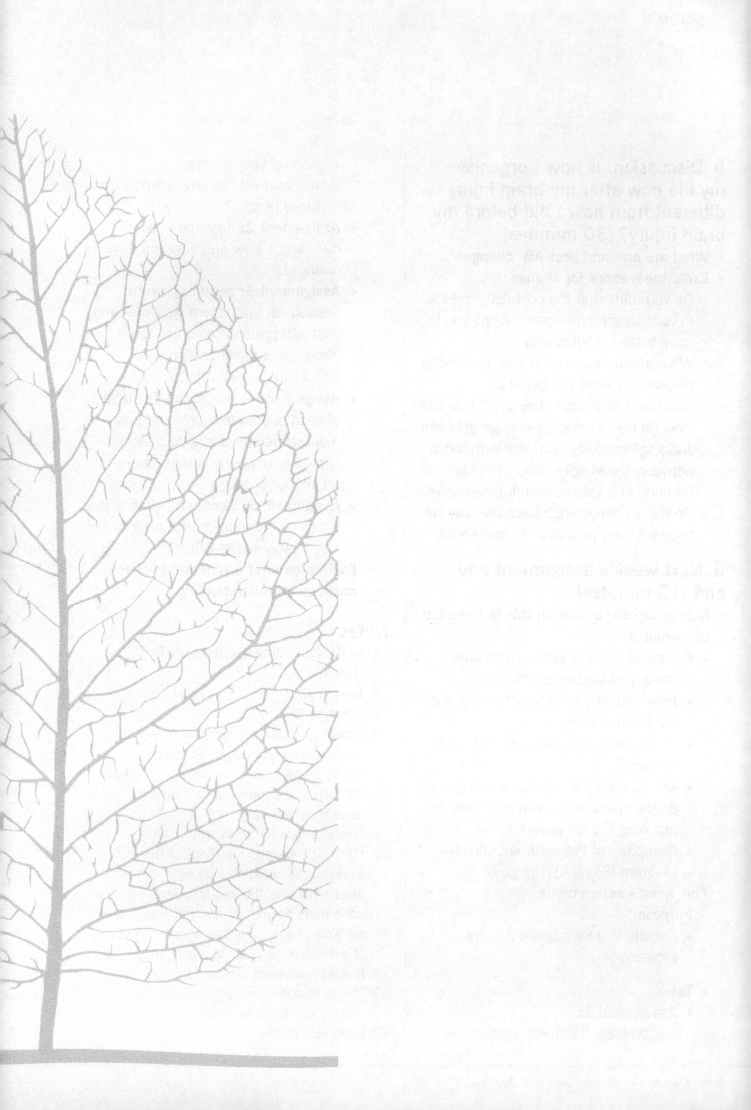

MODULE 2

Exploring change

Introduction to module 2

This module prepares participants for active engagement with therapy. Its central tasks are to

1   Focus on the dysfunctional coping mechanisms participants use to manage the adverse consequences of ABI
2   Demonstrate that dealing with change with different coping strategies may be more effective and probably safer
3   Raise motivation to trial different coping strategies to master post-ABI frame breaking change

The first three of the module's five sessions introduce the CBT constructs of the thought-feeling-behaviour cycle, automatic thoughts and rules and protective behaviours. The fourth session explores the consequences of unexpected, unplanned rule breakdown and the last session invites participants to identify the 'agent' who devises their rules and supporting protective behaviours.

The sessions increasingly rely on the principles of **experiential learning**. They encourage participants to actively engage in the learning experience by reflecting on their actions during group sessions in the here and now and in real life outside the group.

Exercises and assignments function as conduits for experiential learning by promoting curiosity, inquiry and reflection and by helping participants develop solutions to real problems, both as individuals and as a team. The key practitioner objective is to encourage the group to involve itself directly in exercises and assignments, and to reflect, discuss and reflect again on its experiences. In this reiterative way, participants gain a better understanding of the drivers of their actions. This enables them to choose to maintain or to let go of the behaviour.

The concept of choice is an important one because it involves metacognitive processing,[1] which the last session in this module ushers in. Metacognition is the ability to use prior knowledge to plan a strategy, to take necessary steps to solve a problem, to reflect on and to evaluate results, and to modify one's approach as needed. It postulates a two-tier model of interactive thinking.

This consists, first, of on-line, or object-level, processing, and second, of metacognitive processing. On-line, object-level processing involves the appraisal of events as they occur and responding to them immediately, without reflection. The response is not a considered reaction because the demand situation immerses individuals in itself and prevents them from evaluating the reality-base of their cognitions, perceptions and interpretations.

In metacognitive mode, however, individuals do not necessarily accept their on-line processing as true representations of reality. They are able to inhibit their immediate response, to step back, and to reality-test the accuracy of their thoughts, perceptions and attributions. This process of distancing from the object level enables them to think through the demand situation with reference to the reality-base of their memories of experiences, assumptions and beliefs.

I call metacognitive processing the **Watching Self** and believe that the faculty of choice comes into play only in this mode. The Watching Self invites individuals to become aware of the thoughts and emotions they have about their thoughts and emotions, to reflect on them, and to take the necessary steps to regulate their approach as necessary.

I encourage participants to strengthen and develop their Watching Self into their own personal coach and/or therapist. This is especially important in community-based ABI groups. Participants of these groups, unlike their residential counterparts, tend to lack the dedicated support of carers to motivate them to engage with rehabilitation strategies. The Watching Self in community contexts may be the sole agent that drives ABI survivors to genuinely partake in therapeutic endeavours when they are removed from therapy.

The sessions of this module last between 115 and 125 minutes and have a similar structure to those of Module 1 with the exception of Sessions 8, 9, and 10 that are in 5 parts. They begin with a welcome that runs through the key learning points of its predecessor and an overview of the present one. Part 2 facilitates a plenary discussion of the previous session and a joint review of assignments. Part 3 introduces the topic of the day, and Part 4 engages participants in the session's exercise. Part 5 is a plenary discussion of the exercise, and Part 6 sets next week's assignment and closes the session. In Sessions 8, 9 and 10 Part 4 incorporates Part 5.

Each session has a Practitioners' Guide, a Participants' Handout and a Support Workers' Guide. The evaluation scale in the Appendix can be used to rate each session.

Support workers continue to have a key role in the successful running of this module.

How we think impacts how we behave

➤ AIMS AND OVERVIEW

The aims of this session are three-fold:

1 Explore the mechanisms participants deploy to cope with the adverse consequences of change
2 Help participants understand how these mechanisms impact emotions, cognitions and behaviours
3 Examine the life quality that these mechanisms affords them

The session builds on the work of Module 1. It celebrates participants' achievement of the tasks of previous sessions and reinforces their motivation for mastery of the changes resulting from ABI. It congratulates them for learning to become their own 'therapists.' This presages the concept of 'metacognition' introduced in the last session of this module as my Watching Self.[2]

It then initiates the tasks of Module 2 by training participants in the basic CBT tenet of the **thought-feeling-behaviour cycle** and by introducing the concepts of **consequence and outcome**. The session's central objective is to raise participants' awareness of how their thoughts impact their life quality by governing their feelings and their behaviour.

The key techniques that help achieve the aims of this session are guided discovery and Socratic questioning.

➤ PROCESS NOTES

Objectives and tasks

Today's objectives

1 Develop understanding of the link between our thinking and our feelings
2 Develop understanding of the link between our thinking and our behaviour
3 Develop our ability to become aware of the negative consequences of the way we think

Tasks:

1 Welcome participants and set out the purpose and outline of the session [10 minutes]
2 Summarise last week's session and review assignments [20 minutes]
3 Introduce the CBT **thought-feeling-behaviour cycle** and the concepts of **consequence and outcome** [30 minutes]
4 Help participants complete the exercise and facilitate feedback [20 minutes]
5 Lead a discussion on the behavioural consequences and outcomes of their **thought-feeling-behaviour cycles** [30 minutes]
6 Explain next week's assignment and end the session [15 minutes]

Total time: 125 minutes

1 Welcome and introduction [10 minutes]

- **Overview of last module:**
  - **Tasks we accomplished in last module:**
    - ♦ Constructed preference profiles pre- and post-ABI.
    - ♦ Identified differences between pre- and post-ABI preference profiles
    - ♦ Worked through reasons for pre- and post-ABI changes
  - **Processes we deployed to accomplish tasks:**
    - ♦ Self-monitoring
    - ♦ Recall and articulation of experiences
    - ♦ Learning to become our own therapists

How we think impacts how we behave

- **Overview of this module:**
  - **Tasks we will accomplish:**
    - Project to the future
    - Decide if there are any changes we wish to make in ourselves and in our lives
    - Identify the changes we wish to make
  - **Processes for accomplishing these tasks:**
    - Same as in Module 1

2 Summary of last session and assignment review [20 minutes]

- **Last session**
  - Recall and articulation of learned material during previous session
  - Summary of changes participants wish to achieve post-ABI
- **Assignment review**
  - **Examples from previous groups** reveal an improved recognition of post-ABI change, a greater awareness of its adverse effects, and an increased preparedness to bring about a more adaptive adjustment to the post-injury order of life. The results of the first assignment table confirm participants' within-session self-ratings and explanations of the pre- and post-ABI changes for Judging and Perceiving.

    Typical participant statements for the second assignment table include:
    - Brain injury forces us to control things and structure our lives.
    - I grin and bear things now; I used to speak my mind before my injury.
    - I trusted myself to be on top of things before my brain injury. Now I worry I will mess up.
    - I was very structured before my brain injury. Now I don't need to be structured because I don't do anything. I prefer things this way now.
    - I have had to structure things to be able to deal with life. I prepare for everything in advance now.
    - My brain injury caused many changes. I live with them. I am not always aware of them.
    - I feel brain injury has forced me to have a more structured lifestyle. Before my injury, I let things happen more. I don't trust myself now.

    Table 1 shows typical type changes:

Table 1 Typical type changes in one group

	Before ABI	After ABI	Change Yes/No
	MBTI Type	MBTI Type	
1	ISTJ	ISTJ	NO
2	ESFJ	ISTP	YES
3	ESFP	ISTJ	YES
4	ENTP	ISTP	YES
5	ENTP	ISFJ	YES
6	ENFP	ISTJ	YES

Typical change aspirations after ABI include:

* ❖ I want to be an extrovert.
* ❖ I want to be able to rely on my own thinking more.
* ❖ I want to make decisions more on feelings. I want to be able to 'stand my ground' more. I feel people take advantage of me because I can't say no.
* ❖ I miss the 'ego boosts' I used to get when I went to parties and out with friends.
* ❖ I feel safer in my own company. I need to protect myself from criticism so I avoid people. I want to be able to deal with people's criticism better.

* ○ **Present group**
* ○ Two or three participants read out BEFORE/AFTER assignment results; they share with the group how they feel about their post-ABI aspirations and why actualising them would improve their lives. They relate their experiences of the week to the aspirations they wish to actualise.

3 How what I think impacts how I feel and behave [30 minutes]

* • **Discussion:**
* ○ Exploring impact of negative thinking on post-ABI preference change; i.e., Extrovert to Introvert; Perceiving to Judging
* ○ Developing understanding of thought leading to anxiety leading to avoidance behaviour

  'I will mess up' → anxiety → avoidance behaviour → ***'I won't go to the party'***

  * ♦ **Explanation**
* ○ *Thought:* 'I *will* mess up'
* ○ *Feeling:* anxiety
* ○ *Behaviour Consequence:* you don't go to the party

* ○ *Outcome:* You avoid meeting new people; you avoid speaking with people in case you 'mess up'; you lose contact with friends; you don't make any new friends. So what has happened has turned you into an introvert. Outcome has impacted the way you lead your life.
* ○ *Consequence* refers to the results of particular events; *outcome* is the wide-ranging impact of these results upon your lifestyle across the board.

* • Thought-Feeling-Behaviour cycle [Handout pages 4 and 5]:

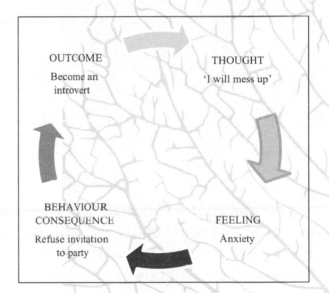

* ○ The diagram links participants' assignment statements of post-ABI adverse change to their behaviour and helps to clarify the relevance of their thoughts to their day-to-day life. Participants are encouraged to cite further examples.

4 Exercise: identifying the outcomes of my thinking [20 minutes]

* • Exercise: Reference to handout, explanation of instructions
* • End exercise: Participants read out their exercise results

How we think impacts how we behave

 Complete the table by giving examples of three of your thoughts in the **THOUGHT** column, stating how each makes you feel in the **FEELING** column, and how you behave as a result of each in the **BEHAVIOURAL CONSEQUENCES** column. Write down the lifestyle outcome in the **OUTCOME** column. The table gives two examples to get you started.

Thought	Feeling	Behavioural Consequences	Outcome
I will mess up	Anxiety	Don't go to the party	Don't meet my friends; don't make new friends
There might be a stampede at the football match	Anxiety	Don't go to football matches any more	Don't go to venues that my friends go to; lose contact with my friends

5 Feedback and discussion: what are the emotional and life-quality outcomes of my negative thinking? [30 minutes]

This exercise illustrates further the operation of the **thought-feeling-behaviour-outcome cycle**. During feedback, participants are encouraged to:

- Identify behavioural consequences of their thinking
- Work out the outcomes of their thought-feeling-behaviour-consequence cycle
- Decide
  - If these outcomes are positive or negative
  - If their mode of thinking is realistic and achievable? i.e., unconditional safety, avoidance of criticism at all times, never 'messing up'

The objectives of the discussion are three-fold:

1 Highlight the maladaptive outcomes of participants' negative thinking
2 Draw attention to the unrealistic, unachievable attributes of this mode of thinking
3 Encourage participants to propose solutions that will improve the adaptive quality of their outcomes

6 Next week's assignment and end [15 minutes]

Assignment recapitulates this session's exercise and discussion. The tables contain examples.

1 Give three examples of your thinking, the feelings each example leads to and the behavioural consequences of each. Then work out the outcome of these **thought-feeling-behaviour cycles**.

2 Identify how you feel about these outcomes

3 State if you wish to change the outcomes of your **thought-feeling-behaviour cycles**, and if yes, then how?

How we think impacts how we behave: automatic thoughts before/after ABI

➤ AIMS AND OVERVIEW

The aim of this session is to lay the foundations of participants' ability to reality-check their interpretation of critical events by developing a considered awareness of their cognitions. The focus continues to be on the impact of thought on behaviour, but the discussion of **Automatic Thoughts** and **Core Beliefs** develops this further and prepares the way for the introduction of the CBT concepts of **Rules**, **Protective** or **Safety Behaviours** and **Metacognitive Processing**.

The session aims to get an 'aha!' feeling from participants by guiding them through the experience of an automatic thought being triggered by an activating event. It uses action learning principles by facilitating a discussion **before** setting out an explanation of automatic thoughts.

The session makes frequent reference to participants' assignment contents to highlight examples of automatic thoughts and to make conceptual explanations relevant and meaningful. It also deploys the therapeutic techniques of Socratic questioning and guided discovery to enable participants to assimilate material arising from their own assignment and exercise results. For example, memory and information-processing difficulties of ABI survivors create in them the automatic thought **'I am not sharp enough [to cope with this anymore]'** when faced with complex tasks such as reviewing the family budget or assembling flat-pack furniture.

Therapeutic interventions occupy the foreground from this point onwards and throughout the programme. Their purpose is to help participants:

1 Unravel the intricacies of their own thinking
2 Arrive at their own answers to the questions that arise as the work progresses
3 Acknowledge and name their answers

It is important not to become involved in prolonged one-on-one therapeutic exchanges but to address interventions to the group as a whole. When a participant appears to be drawing close to discovering and acknowledging an answer to a question, reinforce this attempt by clarifying, by asking the group to share their own examples and by enlisting their help in naming it. Group sharing enriches learning because it makes experiences feel 'real' and relevant for everybody and reinforces group cohesion.

The task remains that of raising awareness of pre- and post-ABI change, but before/after difference comparisons tend to move to the background after this session. This is because it is beyond the scope of this programme to identify and to address any dysfunctional personality propensities that existed before the ABI occurred.

➤ PROCESS NOTES

Objectives and tasks

Objectives:

1 Develop participants' understanding of automatic thoughts
2 Help participants explore the automatic thoughts they have developed after ABI
3 Help participants acknowledge and name the core beliefs which generated them

How we think impacts how we behave: automatic thoughts before/after ABI

Tasks:

1 Welcome participants and set out the purpose and outline of the session [10 minutes]
2 Summarise last week's session and review assignments [20 minutes]
3 Introduce the concept of Automatic Thoughts [30 minutes]
4 Facilitate comparison between pre- and post-ABI automatic thoughts, help participants complete the exercise and facilitate feedback [25 minutes]
5 Introduce the concept of Core Beliefs and lead a discussion drawing examples from the exercise [30 minutes]
6 Explain next week's assignment and end the session [15 minutes]

Total time: 130 minutes

1 Welcome and introduction [10 minutes]
As set out in task list

2 Summary of last session and assignment review [20 minutes]
- Last session
  - The thought-feeling-behaviour-consequence-outcome cycle
  - Negative thoughts lead to negative emotions
  - Negative emotions produce dysfunctional behaviour

- **Assignment review**
  - **Examples from previous groups:** Tables 2 and 3 present typical three-table combined assignment results. They show an effective understanding of the content of the last session

Table 2 Typical combined assignment results of the first two tables of Session 6

Thought	Feeling	Behavioural Consequence	Outcome	Emotion
1 Will not cope with all this information	Anxiety	Leave bills unpaid	Late payment notices	Depressed; disappointed with self
2 Bedrooms are in a mess	Anxiety	Spend time putting order to bedrooms	Leave other household chores undone	Out of control; depressed, anxious
3 Son refuses to accept advice	Anger	Row	Poor relationship	Anxious, depressed
4 I will be late for my appointment	Anxiety	Leave 2 hours early	Leave household chores undone	Angry with self; depressed
5 Shopkeeper ignoring me	Anger	Walk out of shop	Not done shopping for the day	Anxious, depressed

How we think impacts how we behave: automatic thoughts before/after ABI

Table 3 Typical summary Table 3 assignment result of session 6

Outcome	How Can I Improve It
Late payment notices	Have greater confidence in self; deal with the information little by little
Leave other household chores undone	Do chores in order of importance; don't worry about disorder in bedrooms, get kids to sort own bedrooms
Poor relationship	Repeat advice; point out what will happen if he does not follow: 'I will charge you if I make your bed.'
Leave household chores undone	Don't leave two hours early; don't worry about being told off
Not done shopping for the day	Don't know shopkeeper is ignoring me; carry on shopping; repeat question to draw his attention

- **Present group**
  - Two or three participants select and share with group thought-feeling-behaviour-outcome cycles. Material is recorded on flip chart. Group discussion follows.

3 My automatic thoughts after/before ABI [30 minutes]

- Stimulate an intuitive understanding of the immediate, involuntary and fleeting quality of automatic thoughts
- Raise awareness of the differences in quality of automatic thoughts pre- and post-ABI
- Facilitate brief discussion that precedes the description of automatic thoughts[3]
- Refer to participants' assignment scenarios and prompt them to answer the questions:
  - How long did I take to think this thought?
  - Did I think it in long sentences?
  - Did I respond with same automatic thoughts pre-ABI to similar scenarios?

- Description of automatic thoughts:
  - Transient
  - Short and specific
  - Occur extremely rapidly before, during or immediately after the event
  - Occur in the stream of consciousness
  - Do not occur in sentences but may consist of a few key words or images
  - Do not arise from careful thought
  - Do not occur in a logical series of steps such as problem solving
  - They happen involuntarily
  - They are thoughts or visual images that derive from past experience and of which we may not be aware unless we focus our attention on them
  - They are all habitual, plausible and believable. We do not evaluate them but think of them as **factual representations of reality**
- The ABI experience: a critical event that generates both a set of new automatic thoughts and reinforces some old negative ones as a result of accumulating post-ABI life experience

How we think impacts how we behave: automatic thoughts before/after ABI

4 Exercise: my automatic thoughts before/after ABI [25 minutes]

- **Pre-exercise mini discussion:** Are the automatic thoughts recorded in the assignments based on post- or pre-ABI life experience? 'I will mess up; I am incompetent; I am not safe' [5 minutes]

- **Exercise:** in handouts, explanation of instructions, completion of exercise [15 minutes]
- **End Exercise:** a couple of participants read out results of the exercise and these are put on flip chart [5 minutes]

How we think impacts how we behave: automatic thoughts before/after ABI

EXERCISE

Please complete the table by selecting an activating event which you have experienced both after and before your ABI. Identify the immediate automatic thoughts and the feelings that this event produced both after and before your ABI. Rate these feelings from 0 to 5 for their negative quality. A rating of 0 indicates no negative emotion; a rating of 5 indicates maximum negative emotion.

Table 4

After ABI			Before ABI		
Activating Event	Automatic Thought	Feeling Rate From 1 To 5 0 = No Negative Emotion; 5 = Maximum Negative Emotion	Same/Similar Activating Event; Recalled Or Imagined	Automatic Thought	Feeling Rate From 1 To 5 0 = No Negative Emotion; 5 = Maximum Negative Emotion

How we think impacts how we behave: automatic thoughts before/after ABI

5 Exercise discussion: the core beliefs which generate my post-ABI automatic thoughts [30 minutes]

- Discussion
  - Comparison of pre- and post-ABI automatic thoughts and emotion ratings
  - Identification of beliefs underlying these rating-differences, e.g., 'son refuses my advice'; 'shopkeeper is ignoring me'
  - How would you name post-ABI beliefs like 'I am incompetent; I am damaged; I am stupid'? What do they say about the way you see yourself?

- Description of core beliefs
  Core beliefs are memory stores of our experience of our 'self,' of others and of the world. They act as filters for ongoing experience. The ABI experience is not only a critical **activating event** that has generated a set of new automatic thoughts, but it has also stimulated our **mental store of negative core beliefs**. We therefore automatically interpret and judge post-ABI events in their light.

- The ABI experience is a critical event that stimulates negative core beliefs; facilitated discussion

6 Next week's assignment and end [15 minutes]

- Repeat of today's exercise with different activating events
- Identify the post-ABI core beliefs that are the basis of the automatic thoughts associated with the three activating events
- Make a list of your post-ABI core beliefs

How we manage our negative core beliefs: rules and protective behaviours

➤ AIMS AND OVERVIEW

This session introduces the CBT concepts of **Rules** and **Protective** or **Safety Behaviours**. It explores the ways in which participants cope with the critical events that confront them in their day-to-day lives. It has three aims: the first is to create the realisation that the behaviours participants deploy in response to anxiety- or distress-provoking events are in fact coping mechanisms.

The second aim is to raise awareness that these coping mechanisms are part of a safety framework participants have developed that protects them from the painful consequences of their ABI.

The third aim is for them to recognise that the central function of their protective framework is to shield them from their negative core beliefs by preventing their automatic thoughts from surfacing into awareness.

➤ PROCESS NOTES

Objectives and tasks

Objectives:

1 Explore how we manage our negative automatic thoughts and core beliefs
2 Learn about protective behaviours and rules/conditional beliefs

Tasks:

1 Welcome participants and set out the purpose and outline of the session [10 minutes]

2 Summarise last week's session and review assignments [20 minutes]
3 How we manage our negative automatic thoughts and core beliefs: discussion and exercise [35 minutes]
4 Introduce and explain the concepts of protective behaviours and rules/conditional beliefs [15 minutes]
5 Lead a discussion drawing examples from the exercise [25 minutes]
6 Explain next week's assignment and end the session [15 minutes]

Total Time: 120 Minutes

1 Welcome and introduction [10 minutes]

As set out in task list

2 Summary of last session and assignment review [20 minutes]

- **Last session**
  - Activating events produce immediate negative thoughts which lead to negative emotions
  - Core beliefs are the source of automatic thoughts
  - ABI experience creates negative and painful core beliefs

- **Assignment review**
  - **Examples from previous groups:** Tables 5–7 display typical summarised assignment results

How we manage our negative core beliefs: rules and protective behaviours

Table 5 Typical post- and pre-ABI comparisons

Post-ABI			Pre-ABI	
Activating Event	**Automatic Thought**	**Negative Feeling Rating** **0–5**	**Automatic Thought**	**Negative Feeling Rating** **0–5**
Daughter did not ask for help	Thinks I am not up to it; I have been replaced	Depression 5	It's up to her; am here if she needs me	Nil
Invited to large music venue	Won't cope with crowd; will have another ABI	Anxiety 5	Great	Nil
Make presentation at gathering	Will mess up; they will think me stupid	Anxiety 5	Hope I will be ok	Anxiety 2
Person did not give way on pavement	No respect for physically disabled	Anger 5	Same as post-ABI	Irritation 3
Shopper collided with me	Smash his face in	Anger 5	Why can't people be more careful?	Irritation 2
Argument with spouse	Treats me like a child; can't get anything right	Depression, anger, 5	Oh not again	Irritation 2

Table 6 Typical Post-ABI core beliefs

Activating Event	Core Belief
Daughter did not ask for help	I am not needed I am worthless I am not sharp I am not respected I don't trust myself I don't trust others
Invited to large music venue	I am not safe I am not in control; not in charge I am at risk
Make presentation at gathering	I am not as good as I was I am not as quick as I was
Person did not give way on pavement	I am faulty goods I am weak I am not safe
Shopper collided with me	The world treats me like sh#t
Argument with spouse	I am useless I am worthless

How we manage our negative core beliefs: rules and protective behaviours

Table 7 Typical post-ABI core belief list

Core Belief List
1 I am not needed
2 I am worthless
3 I am not sharp
4 I am not respected
5 I don't trust myself
6 I don't trust others
7 I am not safe
8 I am not in control
9 I am not in charge
10 I am at risk
11 I am not as good as I was
12 I am not as quick as I was
13 I am faulty goods
14 I am weak
15 The world treats me like sh#t
16 I am useless

- **Present group**
  - Two or three participants select a couple of activating events from their assignments and share with the group the core beliefs associated with them
  - Two or three participants read out their list of core beliefs. These are noted on the flip chart

- Participants help select core beliefs held in common by all and discuss their negative, painful qualities

3 How we manage our negative core beliefs: exercise [35 minutes]

- Dual focus: Help participants realise that the behaviours they deploy in response to activating events are in fact coping mechanisms; pave the way for the introduction of rules/conditional beliefs and protective behaviours
- Pre-exercise mini-group discussion [10 minutes]
  - Examination of participants' behaviours in session 6 assignments and of their explanations of post-ABI MBTI preference changes; most relevant are changes in Extroversion/Introversion and Judging/Perceiving
  - Participants understand and articulate that their responses to activating events represent their way of coping with their demands

- Exercise [15 minutes]: In handouts, explanation of instructions
- Post Exercise [10 minutes]: participants read out exercise results and these are put on flip chart
- Group discussion and review of results

How we manage our negative core beliefs: rules and protective behaviours

Exercise

Please complete the table by selecting an actual activating event. Identify the immediate automatic thought and its underlying core belief. Then describe what you actually did.

Table 8

Activating Event	Automatic Thought	Core Belief	Behavioural Consequence

How we manage our negative core beliefs: rules and protective behaviours

4 Conditional beliefs or rules and protective behaviours: discussion [25 minutes]

- **Purpose:** first, to steer participants to discover, acknowledge and name the rules and supporting protective behaviours they deploy to cope with post-ABI life demands; second, to function as a rehearsal for completion of this session's assignment

- **Explanation**
  - **Conditional Beliefs/Rules**

    It is unusual for people who have a core belief that they are flawed to think that they are 'flawed' *all the time*, because such people usually have memories which conflict with this belief.

    For example, we do not feel worthless or incompetent when a family member or friend shows us appreciation of what we have done for them, or when we have worked hard at a task and completed it successfully.

    We therefore develop **conditional beliefs**, or **rules**, which we think of as 'if-then' statements. They are conditional, because we do not know that they are true; we assume they are true.

    For example, if we feel good about ourselves when a family member expresses appreciation of our help, we might develop a rule that reads, *'If people show me appreciation, then I might be okay,'* or *'If people don't show me any appreciation then I am worthless.'*

    If we feel good about ourselves when we complete a task successfully, then we are likely to develop a rule that reads something like, *'If I succeed in everything I do, I might not be incompetent'* or, *'If I am less than always successful, then I'm incompetent.'*

    These rules ensure that we behave in certain ways so as to keep the negative belief 'I am worthless' or 'I am incompetent' away from our immediate awareness. They force us to behave in certain ways. For example, we feel obliged to over-work at tasks to be successful at them, or to always please people to feel competent or good about ourselves.

  - **Protective Behaviours**

    This framework of core beliefs and rules is supported by certain **PROTECTIVE or SAFETY BEHAVIOURS**. These protective behaviours protect us from the activation of negative automatic thoughts and core beliefs. An example of a safety behaviour is when we behave in ways which lead others to show us their appreciation of what we have done. The appreciation we seek and receive to stop our negative thought *'I am incompetent'* from surfacing and so shields us from our negative core belief *'I am worthless.'*

  - **Summary**

    Conditional beliefs are 'if-then' statements: conditional, because we do not know that they are true; we assume they are true. Protective behaviours support our rules and shield us from our negative core beliefs.

How we manage our negative core beliefs: rules and protective behaviours

- **Discussion**
  - Participants link their behaviour consequences from the exercise to protective behaviours
  - Participants generate more examples of their own protective behaviours
  - Participants identify the rules that their protective behaviours support

5 Next week's assignment and end [15 minutes]

This session has three assignments:

1 Identification of automatic thoughts underlying core beliefs and protective behaviours in response to activating events

2 Description of the rules that are supported by these protective behaviours

3 Construction of a list of post-ABI rules in response to negative core beliefs

What happens when post-ABI rules break down?

➤ AIMS AND OVERVIEW

This session aims to convey to participants that their post-ABI safety framework of rules and protective behaviours is dysfunctional. It achieves this aim by gradually exposing participants to the maladaptive aspects of this framework through exercise and discussion.

Maladaptive outcomes are consistent with expectation of the post-ABI adjustment of survivors who partake in therapeutic groups. However, the level of impairment in adjustment that some ABI survivors' outcomes suggest will exceed the therapeutic scope of CBT work in group format. These cases will require referral to different, more intensive treatment formats.

There is little theoretic content in this session. Participants do the work themselves through the application of experiential learning principles and the help of guided discovery.

➤ PROCESS NOTES

Objectives and tasks

This session's objectives are for participants to explore:

1 If all their post-ABI rules are sensible, attainable and realistic
2 If they can uphold all their post-ABI rules at all times
3 What is likely to happen when their post-ABI rules break down

Tasks:

1 Welcome participants, set out the purpose and outline of the session [10 minutes]

2 Summarise last week's session and review assignments [20 minutes]
3 Run a joint group exercise to test the first two session objectives: 'Are all post-ABI rules sensible, attainable and realistic?' [40 minutes]
4 Facilitate a discussion to test the third session objective: 'What happens when post-ABI rules break down?' [30 minutes]
5 Explain next week's assignment and end the session [15 minutes]

Total time: 115 minutes

1 Welcome and introduction [10 minutes]

As set out in task list

2 Summary of last session and assignment review [20 minutes]

- **Last session**
  - Behaviour consequences are coping mechanisms
  - Rules and protective behaviours help us manage our negative core beliefs
  - Rules keep our negative core beliefs away from our immediate awareness
  - Our protective behaviours are the behaviour consequences of our Thought-Feeling-Behaviour-Outcome cycle
  - Protective behaviours support and enforce our rules to keep negative core beliefs away from immediate awareness

- **Assignment review**
  - **Examples from previous groups:** Tables 9–10 display typical summarised assignment results.

What happens when post-ABI rules break down?

Table 9 Coping with activating events

Activating Event	Automatic Thought	Core Belief	Protective Behaviour	Rule
Dropped whole dinner plate on kitchen floor	I can't even manage this	I am crap	Don't let anyone in kitchen; clear up mess without anyone noticing	If I do not let anyone see me mess up, they will not see I am crap
Bought set of faulty scales but lost receipt	I'll be laughed out of court if I take it back	I am stupid I am incompetent I am faulty goods	Say nothing; buy another set	If I avoid confrontation I will not lose face/look silly
Buying shirt with wife who rushed me	She won't even make this time for me	I am worthless I am a burden	Gave in to pressure; let her decide what I should buy	If I keep quiet I will keep harmony
Car wouldn't start	Sure car is OK; it's me	Can't think straight I am incompetent	Asked neighbour to check car	If others agree with me then I am OK
Handed in mobile phone for cash; offered less than advertised	I am being duped; shop assistant is riding roughshod over me	I am stupid I am small I am a sucker They are all jumped-up thieving gits	Told them to shove it and walked out	If I show anger they will respect me more; I will appear strong

Table 10 Post-ABI core belief rule list

Core Beliefs	Rules
I am crap	If I do not let anyone see me mess up, they will not see I am crap
I am faulty goods	If I avoid confrontation I will not lose face/look silly
I am worthless I am a burden	If I keep quiet I will keep harmony If I keep quiet I won't be criticised
Can't think straight I am incompetent	If others agree with me then I am OK
I am small I am a sucker They are all jumped-up thieving gits	If I show anger they will respect me more If I shout I will appear strong

What happens when post-ABI rules break down?

- **Present group**
  - Participants recall and articulate material that they have learned during the previous session
  - Two or three participants select a couple of activating events from their assignments and share with the group the protective behaviours they used to manage them
  - Two or three participants read out their list of core beliefs and related rules. These are noted on the flip chart
  - Participants help select the rules they hold in common and discuss if and when they are useful
  - Practitioners steer participants to begin to question the adaptive quality of their rules and protective behaviours

3 Are all post-ABI rules sensible, attainable and realistic: can we uphold them at all times? [40 minutes]

- **Group Exercise**
  - **Objective:** demonstrate that
    - Rules cannot be upheld at all times because they are not sensible and realistic
    - Rules do not enduringly protect us from our negative core beliefs
  - **Process:** Group exercise
    - Participants work as a team[4]
    - Participants express views and share their experiences
    - Exercise diagram is already on flip chart

Activating Event	Automatic Thought	Protective Behaviours	Life Rule

- **Instructions:** Participants jointly select an activating event from their assignments which represents a common experience that they have all shared. Participants complete the exercise figure which is already on the flip chart. Alternatively, they can complete the exercise tables below

Consequence	Emotion	Lifestyle Outcome

- **Examples from previous groups:** The next pages present two typical examples. The first demonstrates the wide-ranging aftermath of an unexpected sudden rule break, and the second shows the negative cognitive, emotional and lifestyle outcomes of adhering to a dysfunctional rule.
- **End Exercise Discussion:**
  - What are the consequences of upholding this rule?
  - What are the lifestyle outcomes of upholding this rule?
  - What are the emotional consequences of upholding this rule?
  - Can I uphold this rule at all times?
  - Does this rule shield me from becoming aware of my negative core beliefs?
- **Exercise Conclusion:** All rules are not sensible, attainable and realistic; we cannot uphold them at all times

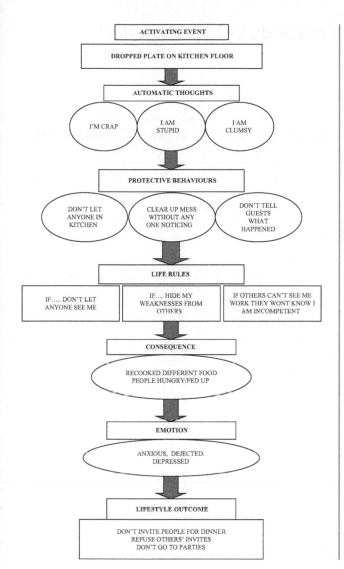

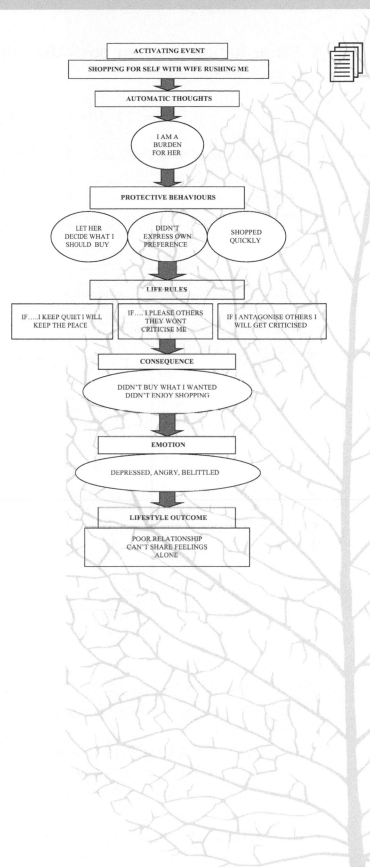

4 What happens when post-ABI rules break down? [30 minutes]
• **Reasons for rule break**

Table 11 The maladaptive quality of some life rules

• Unrealistic standards/demands	If I do everything perfectly then people will not criticise me If I prepare for every eventuality then I will be safe
• Conflict with and contrary to human emotion and behaviour	If I always please people they will not disapprove of me If I hide my feelings then people won't know I am upset
• Poor coping success	If I set out 2 hours early then I will not be late [but traffic jam thwarts on-time arrival]
• Self-perpetuating vicious circle quality	If I try harder it will work next time

• **Rule break vicious circle**

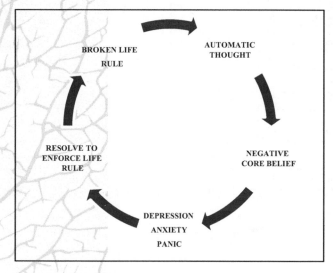

BROKEN LIFE RULE

AUTOMATIC THOUGHT

NEGATIVE CORE BELIEF

DEPRESSION ANXIETY PANIC

RESOLVE TO ENFORCE LIFE RULE

Figure 2.1 Rule break vicious circle

When rules break in uncontrolled situations in unanticipated ways, the after-effects seem chaotic, unmanageable and painful. In contrast, when we plan and engineer rule breaks, we anticipate and prepare ourselves to cope with the consequence.

5 Next week's assignment and end [15 minutes]
• What are my key life rules? What protective behaviours follow from my life rules?
• What happens when my life rules break down?
• Why have my rules broken down?
• What did I do when my rules broke down } (Assignment Table 3)?

Someone to watch over me

➤ AIMS AND OVERVIEW

This is the last session of this module. Its aim is to engage participants' motivation and personality resources to master the frame-breaking changes that have impacted their post-ABI life order by actively trialling the therapeutic strategies that Module 3 will set out.

The session therefore borrows from metacognitive therapy,[5] the two-tier model of information processing comprising on-line, object-level processing and metacognitive processing. It encourages participants to strengthen and to develop their Watching Self into their own personal coach and/or therapist.

This session's central focus is on stimulating participants to co-opt the Watching Self to motivate them to genuinely engage with the therapeutic strategies that the final module of the program will set out.

➤ PROCESS NOTES

Objectives and tasks

Objectives: We will learn

1 How we process critical events
2 Who watches over us when we face critical events
3 How we can learn to be more effective in managing our emotions and behaviour in the face of critical events

Tasks:

1 Welcome; set out the purpose and outline of the session [10 minutes]
2 Summarise last week's session and review assignments [20 minutes]
3 Introduce and explain the Watching Self: **'How we process a critical event'** [30 minutes]

4 Run a group exercise to raise awareness of and to strengthen the Watching Self: **'Someone to watch over me'** [15 minutes]
5 Facilitate a group discussion that aligns the Watching Self to therapeutic goals: **'Managing our emotions and behaviour when faced with a critical event'** [30 minutes]
6 Explain next week's assignment and end the session [15 minutes]

Total time: 120 minutes

1 Welcome [10 minutes]

• As set out in task list
• Reminder: this is the last session of the module. It helps make an entry to Module 3, in which we learn to master the adverse consequences of ABI by actively engaging with therapeutic initiatives. The time therefore is right for us to ask, 'Who is watching over me?' We explore answers to this question.

2 Summary of last session and assignment review [20 minutes]

• **Last session**
  ○ We cannot uphold all our rules at all times because they are not realistic, sensible or achievable
  ○ Our rules fail to protect us as we intend them to do because they break down unexpectedly in uncontrolled situations
  ○ Rules break down because they:
    ♦ Place unattainable demands upon us
    ♦ Conflict with and oppose our human emotions and behaviour
    ♦ Have a poor success record
    ♦ Have a self-perpetuating vicious circle quality
  ○ When rules break down unexpectedly, they lead to unmanageable and painful consequences

- **Assignment review**
  - **Examples from previous groups:** Tables 12–13 set out typical assignment results
  - **Present group:** Participants recall and articulate material that they have learned during the previous session. During this section's discussion, practitioners highlight that rule breakdown occurred unexpectedly because participants' rules were unrealistic and unachievable and therefore could not be upheld in all situations. Participants are encouraged to articulate these reasons with reference to their assignments. They receive help to express how they coped with the ensuing chaos of rule breakdown. How did they deal with their feelings and the situation?

Typical Assignment Examples

Table 12 What are my key life rules? What protective behaviours follow from my life rules?

Participants	Life Rules	Protective Behaviours
1	• Avoid taking centre stage • Hide my weaknesses from others • Avoid public/crowded environments • Be always prepared in case I lose control	• Refuse invitations/parties • Don't allow people in my kitchen • Don't go out in rush hour • Leave well before time for appointments
2	• Cut myself off; live in a bubble • Avoid stress • Be always prepared for the worst	• Don't go to pubs/gatherings • Put bills to one side • Overrehearse tasks in advance
3	• Don't show my emotions • Avoid criticism • Others must think well of me	• Don't watch sad films • Check out my decisions with others • Check that I have done my best
4	• Be always prepared • Remain focused on what might go wrong • Always think ahead so all aspects are covered	• Avoid situations I cannot control • Avoid all distraction • Stick to daily structure
5	• Do everything perfectly • Make myself useful to show I am worthwhile • Plan all I do in advance • Keep harmony at all costs	• Practise in advance everything I say and do • Ask questions about everything to do things right • Don't get involved with unexpected events/friends • Don't disagree/argue

Someone to watch over me

Table 13 What happens when my protective behaviours break down?

Participants	Activating Event	Broken Rule	Why Has My Rule Broken Down?	What Did I Do/ Feel When My Rule Broke Down?
1	Took food out of the oven before it was cooked when buzzer sounded	Make yourself useful to show your worth; ask questions about everything	Made an assumption that buzzer meant food was ready without asking first	Worthless; useless; upset; said nothing
2	Dropped plate on kitchen floor Was late for GP appointment	Hide my weaknesses from others Be always prepared in case I lose control	Allowed friends in kitchen Arrived half an hour late because bus was late	I'm crap, clumsy Missed my appointment; rubbish at time management; should have left earlier
3	Went shopping and an old man pushed past me	Cut myself off; stay in my bubble; avoid contact with people	Asked to do shopping for someone else and could not refuse	Angry; just managed to stop myself from hitting him; thought 'it's going to be a nightmare'
4	Accepted invite to music concert	Be always prepared; avoid situations I can't control	Brother insisted; could not refuse	Anxious, panic; I am not in control of my own safety; will have another ABI
5	Did a presentation test	Avoid criticism Don't put self on centre stage Focus on what might go wrong	Accepted and took risk, didn't think ahead	Anxious; worried people will think I am no good

3 How we process a critical event: our Watching Self [30 minutes]

- **Overview of on-line processing:** explanation of Figure 2.1 [on flip chart in advance of session]

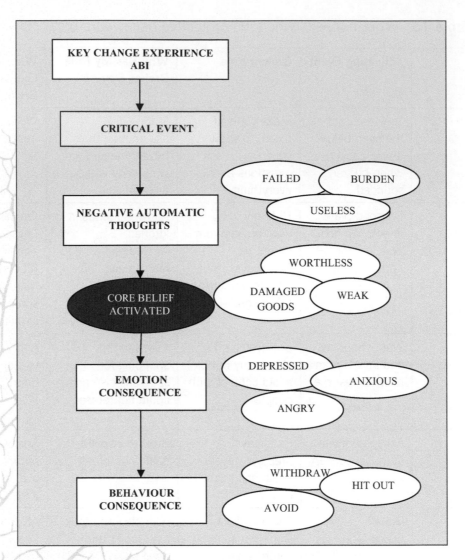

Figure 2.2 Processing critical events

The figure describes the activation of negative automatic thoughts and underlying dysfunctional core beliefs during an on-going unsuccessful encounter with a post-ABI critical event in which the individual is immersed.[6] The thoughts and beliefs are the product of this unsuccessful encounter. They are inflexible, unmodulated and accepted as truths about the self, others and the world.

• **Co-opting the Watching Self:** explanation of Figure 2.3 [on flip chart in advance of session]

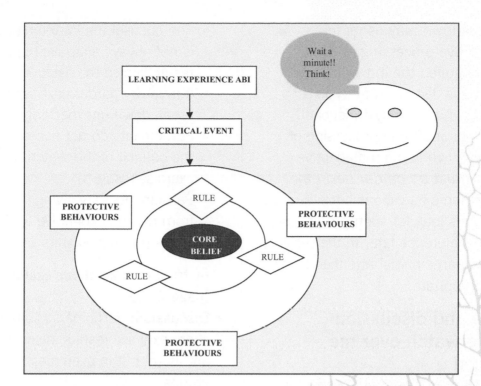

Figure 2.3 Brings into play protective strategies in the form of 'if/then' assumptions that protect individuals from unforeseen consequences. The critical event activates protective behaviours whose role is to support the rules that shield from the painful awareness of negative core beliefs.

The central question for participants here is, Who is the agent that mobilises these strategies as a shield against the pain of perceived failure?

Guided discovery steers participants to

- Realise that the agent is their very own Watching Self.[7]
- Understand that the Watching Self
  - Gives time to self-appraise in relation to the critical event
  - Creates a problem-solving set by allowing distancing from emotional turmoil

- **Discussion:**
  - Are participants able to recognise themselves in this process?
  - How did they come to discover their rules?
  - Were there, for example, any experiences in which these rules achieved their purpose?

- **Points to note:**
  - The maladaptive qualities of participants' rules and protective behaviours do not detract from the importance of the Watching Self in harnessing and maintaining therapeutic engagement. The purpose here is to raise awareness of its presence and function. It is the task of Module 3 to convert dysfunctional metacognitive solutions into effective coping strategies.

Someone to watch over me

○ Rule breakdown may usher in metacognitive processing. If panic has not engulfed the individual, then processing is distanced from object level, even if it were dysfunctional. An example of off-line processing of rule breakdown is the maladaptive resolve '*I must try harder next time*' that represents its vicious circle quality. Practitioners look for such processing, note it for reference later in the session and draw participants' attention to it when appropriate.

4 Exercise and discussion: someone to watch over me [45 minutes]

- **Examples from previous groups** reveal:
- ○ Some participants have rudimentary awareness of the Watching Self [exercise results 1, 3, 4, 6]
- ○ The counsel the Watching Self gives is not always adaptive [e.g., exercise result 1; also the dysfunctional resolve 'I must try harder next time' when rules break down unexpectedly]
- ○ Participants do not necessarily heed the council of the Watching Self [e.g., exercise result 6]
- ○ Participants may swing back and forth from the metacognitive to the object levels [exercise results 1 and 6]

- **Instructions: as above exercise table [page 211]**
- **Discussion:** Participants volunteer to share exercise results; discussion topics are as set out in examples from previous groups

Someone to watch over me

Exercise sample results 2: someone to watch over me [15 minutes]

Complete the table below by filling the appropriate columns. Think of an activating event, the automatic thoughts it activated and the rules linked to these thoughts. Then try to remember if your Watching Self spoke to you at all to help you manage the situation. If it did not, then write 'NO' in the Watching Self column. State the outcome of the event and the emotions you felt as a result.

Activating Event	Automatic Thoughts	Rule	Did Your Watching Self Speak? What Did It Say?	Outcome	Emotional Consequence
1 Asked GP to visit; he came and asked me why I wanted the visit; he hadn't read my notes	He is showing me up; he is making a fool of me	If I show I am angry people will respect me	Apply rule	Showed angry; told him he should've looked at notes before coming; he examined me	Anger; he is incompetent, I am a fool, everybody is against me
2 Was late for group because of traffic	I will be told off; I will not be able to catch up; I will have to do extra work	I must be as good as I was before ABI	No	I was not told off; everything was ok	Relief
3 Son asked for help with maths homework	I am crap, he is doing it on purpose to make me feel small	Hide my weaknesses	I am being defensive; what is important is to feel ok in my own skin	Helped him	It was not too bad
4 Asked to demonstrate leg press at the gym	Am no good at it; will look foolish; not in control	Don't put myself in the limelight	It doesn't matter if I break the rule here	Broke the rule; it went very well	Pleased with self
5 Alarm failed to go off; was late waking up and going shopping	I am useless; a burden; people waiting	Make myself useful to show my worth	No	Was late	Upset
6 Daughter took my hairbrush away with her	She is winding me up; she does it on purpose	Do not show my feelings	Don't send angry text; deal with it when she returns	We had a shouting match and I grounded her	I felt angry and disappointed

5 Assignment and end [15 minutes]

- **Aim of assignment:** to facilitate consolidation of this session's learning material; to sharpen awareness of the Watching Self
- **Content:** repeat of this session's exercise and aims

Notes

1 Wells (2002, 2007, 2009)
2 This is the way I describe metacognition to my patients.
3 In line with **Action learning principles**

4 Groups of up to seven participants can work together as a unit. Groups larger than seven participants will require splitting into syndicates of four participants each.
5 Wells (2002, 2007, 2009); Fisher and Wells (2009)
6 This is an on-line, object level experience.
7 A working analogy is the way people manage a tummy upset. At the object level, they experience flatulence, pain and sickness. If the digestive problems continue, then, at the metacognitive level, the Watching Self distances them from the discomfort and pain, assesses the symptoms and counsels consultation with a medical professional.

MODULE 3

Mastering change

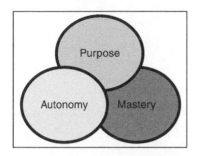

Practitioners' introduction to module

This last module of the programme actively engages in therapy with the application of imaginary and real-life exposure to critical events. Relaxation training is the central tool of imaginary exposure, and behavioural experiments are the method of in-vivo exposure. Group process continues to rely on the Watching Self to motivate and guide participants.

The module has four key aims:

- Develop acknowledgment and acceptance of post-ABI adverse changes
- Build belief in self-efficacy through a sense of enactive attainment over events that affect day-to-day life
- Enable generalisation of self-efficacy to other situations in which performance was debilitated by post-ABI negative core beliefs and dysfunctional rules
- Empower gain of mastery over post-ABI life order

The module's central precepts derive from the research findings of Cicerone et al.[1] that perceived self-efficacy, based on activity-related satisfaction, makes the most significant contribution to the global life satisfaction of ABI survivors.

We continue the scaffolding work of Module 2 with successive sessions building on the learning experience of their predecessors. There are five sessions. Session 11 prepares the group to trial voluntary rule breaks in their day-to-day lives. Session 12 motivates participants to trial real-life exposure to critical events with the application of relaxation together with imaginary exposure. Sessions 13 and 14 focus on goal achievement and experience of personal control to modify negative core beliefs and to let go of dysfunctional rules. The final session reframes the ABI experience as a benchmark whose mastery withstands comparison with answering most of life's other critical demands.

The sessions last between 115 and 135 minutes and have a similar structure to those of the previous two modules. They begin with a welcome that runs through the key learning points of their predecessors and an overview of the present one. Part 2 facilitates a plenary discussion of the previous session and a joint review of assignments. Part 3 introduces the topic of the day and part 4 engages participants in discussion of the session's topic or exercise. Part 5 is a plenary discussion of learning gains, and Part 6 sets next week's assignment and closes the session.

Session 11 is only in 4 parts because of an extended part 3. Sessions 14 has only 5 parts because joint group exercises make a separate feedback section superfluous.

Each session has a Practitioners' Guide, a Participants' Handout and a Support Workers' Guide. The evaluation scale in the Appendix can be used to rate each session.

Support workers continue to have a key role in the successful running of this module.

Breaking rules voluntarily

➤ AIMS AND OVERVIEW

In this first session of Module 3, our aim is to prepare the group to actively trial voluntary rule breaks in their day-to-day lives. This two-step process involves sharpening participants' awareness of:

1 The difference between 'on-line' and 'metacognitive processing' before and during critical events
2 Their Watching Self and engaging in dialogue with it

During discussion of metacognitive processing, some participants may attribute reduction of negative emotions to dealing with imaginary scenarios, as opposed to real, critical events.

In response to this counter, practitioners must invite participants to generate yet more of their own solutions to managing actual critical demands. How should they go about coping with these demands in reality? Could the solution be, for example, to take *'bite-sized chunks of the elephant'*? Could it be to prepare in advance for possible negative outcomes by mentally rehearsing their various components?

The session's intent is to convey to participants that they are their own Watching Self. They are the repository of their self-knowledge, their judgment and the solutions to the problems they face.

➤ PROCESS NOTES

Objective and tasks

Objective:

Become aware of and listen to our Watching Self when faced with critical events

Tasks:

1 Welcome and introduction [10 minutes]
2 Summary of last session and assignment review [20 minutes]
3 Become aware of and listen to our Watching Self when faced with critical events [70 minutes]
  ○ Exercise 1: breaking the rules 'cold' before or during a critical event: consequences [15 minutes]
  ○ Discussion exercise 1 [20 minutes]
  ○ Exercise 2: breaking rules voluntarily with the support of Watching Self before or during a critical event: consequences [15 minutes]
  ○ Discussion exercise 2 [20 minutes]
4 Next week's assignment and end [15 minutes]

Total time: 115 minutes

1 Welcome and introduction [10 minutes]

As in previous sessions

2 Summary of last session and assignment review [20 minutes]

• Recall of previous session:
  ○ When we appraise critical events without evaluating the reality-base of what we think about them, they generate in us negative automatic thoughts and negative emotions
  ○ Our Watching Self protects us from painful critical events by helping us to distance ourselves from them and to think them through
  ○ By distancing ourselves from critical events, our Watching Self enables us to develop strategies that protect us by keeping our automatic thoughts at bay and shielding us from our negative core beliefs

Breaking rules voluntarily

- ○ Our rules are our protective strategies
- ○ However, sometimes the rules that we develop with the help of our Watching Self are not realistic and achievable and we cannot adhere to them
- ○ At other times, we ignore the advice of our Watching Self because we do not trust it
- ○ We then end up immersed in the critical event and face to face with our automatic thoughts and core beliefs

- **Assignment review**
  - ○ **Examples from previous groups:** Table 1 sets out typical assignment results. These reveal that some participants appear to have taken note of the counsel of their Watching Self and some have not [Results 2, 3, 6 vs. 1, 4, 5]
  - ○ **Present group**
    - ♦ Participants recall and articulate material that they have learned during the previous session
    - ♦ Participants share and discuss the content of both assignments with the group
  - ○ **Discussion points**
    - ♦ Positive emotional consequences such as 'relief' are likely to reinforce negative outcomes [Example Assignment 1]
    - ♦ Negative outcomes can sometimes lead to negative emotional consequences [Example Assignments 4, 5, 6]
    - ♦ The advice of the Watching Self can be maladaptive [Example Assignment 6]

Table 1 Typical assignment results for Session 10

Activating Event	Automatic Thoughts	Rule	Did Your Watching Self Speak? What Did It Say?	Outcome	Emotional Consequence
1 Catch the bus 40 mins early for GP appointment	I will be late I will miss the bus	Always give self ample time to get there and settle down	You could leave only 20 mins early, you would still be on time.	Left 40 mins early, arrived in plenty of time	Relief
2 Dropped fork at the restaurant	I am stupid I am an idiot I am clumsy	Hide my weaknesses	Many people drop things by accident; you can get yourself another fork	No one noticed; got another fork	It was OK

(Continued)

Breaking rules voluntarily

Table 1 (Continued)

Activating Event	Automatic Thoughts	Rule	Did Your Watching Self Speak? What Did It Say?	Outcome	Emotional Consequence
3 Told wife I would like to leave half-an-hour later for appointment	There will be a row Won't agree Will be overruled We'll be late	Keep harmony; please others Don't let them think you a burden	Making a suggestion is not a row; 20 miles on motorway in 30 minutes is logical; not rush hour; can still accept her timing if no agreement	Wife agreed; we were not late	Surprise
4 Going to pick up cat from stranger by myself	Will not be able to get my words out It will go wrong Will be clumsy	Hide your weaknesses from others Don't put self centre-stage	Have picked cat up from others before, Nothing went wrong; all I need to say is hello and thank you	Went with mum	Disappointed with self
5 Going to a show that friend has organised in a place that I have never been before (I have had no input)	I might have got the wrong day I might be late and miss show There might be a stampede	Keep control of situations Do not put self in danger Avoid risky places	No	Didn't go	Disappointment Let down self and friend
6 Start a conversation with a group of people I don't know	Will get confused Lose thread of what is said; they will think I am thick Will feel a fool Will need to go and hide somewhere	Do not put self where people judge me Avoid situations that tax memory	You can't rehearse in advance; don't know what will be said	Did not do it	Felt safer but sad as not as sharp as I was pre-ABI

3 Become aware of our Watching Self when faced with critical events [70 minutes]

- **Purpose of section:**
  - Demonstrate that
    - ◆ Automatic thoughts and consequent negative emotions occur primarily when we construe events without evaluating the reality-base of our cognitions, perceptions and interpretations

Breaking rules voluntarily

- ♦ The negative emotional consequences of such processing makes us feel as though we were losing control
  - ○ Develop the ability to step back and to reality-test the accuracy of our thoughts and interpretations to think through critical events and evolve solutions to the problems they pose
  - ○ Recognise the Watching Self as the agent that enables us to step back from events and reality-test our cognitions and interpretations
  - ○ Train in visualisation of critical events and their consequences in preparation for the next session

- • **Exercise 1: breaking rules 'cold' during a critical event: consequences [15 minutes]**
  - ○ **Instructions**
    - ♦ Actively engage in imagining a critical event scenario in which you are unable to apply your rule. Imagine vividly what would happen and how you would feel. [1 minute]
    - ♦ Record the scenes you have visualised on Table 1 / Exercise 1[2] [15 minutes]
    - ♦ Table 2 offers typical examples
  - ○ **Discussion [20 minutes]**
    - ♦ Vivid description of visualised images of 'palpitating, shaking, fainting'
    - ♦ Do these images reflect fear of loss of control?
    - ♦ 'Engulfing' nature of on-line processing
    - ♦ Anticipated nature of fear of loss of control
    - ♦ Avoidance as the key dysfunctional rule and protective behaviours
    - ♦ Appraisal of advantages and disadvantages of adhering to rules

Table 2 Typical examples from previous groups

Rule	Activating Event	Automatic Thought	Rule Break Emotional Consequence
1 Always give self/leave a lot more time than needed	Friend invites for lunch in another town	Will be late getting daughter from school Will miss bus back Traffic will be bad Bus will not arrive Will be pushing it for time	Panic; disaster
2 Do not put self in situations where I appear different from other people; hide my weaknesses	Go to library to ask about taking out talking books	Wish I didn't need them They will think I can't read They will think I am stupid	Apprehension; shame; depressed
3 Don't put self in situations that make demands on memory	Group asks me to buy cake for next week without writing it down	I will forget They will feel sorry for me I will let them all down	Anxiety; shame; depressed

(Continued)

Table 2 (Continued)

Rule	Activating Event	Automatic Thought	Rule Break Emotional Consequence
4 Hide my weaknesses; hide my emotions	Cook dinner for my boyfriend in front of him	Will be crap Food will be awful Will look like an idiot Will be useless Will not cope with pressure	Panic; shame
5 Avoid situations I cannot control Don't risk being made a fool of	Ring up opticians to find out results of eye test to see if I can drive again	Will not have passed Be a bad result Just my luck Why me? Will never be independent	Anxiety; shame; depressed; what's the point?

- **Exercise 2: Breaking rules voluntarily with the support of Watching Self before or during a critical event: consequences [15 minutes]**
  - **Instructions**
    - Please now actively think of the same critical event but imagine yourself thinking it through and discussing it with your Watching Self as it happens. Please ensure your visualisation of the scenario and of your conversation with your Watching Self is very vivid, as if the whole scene were happening here and now
    - Complete the table in Exercise 2.[3] [1 minute imagination time; 14 minutes recording time]
    - Table 3 offers typical examples from previous groups

  - **Discussion [20 minutes]**
    - Description of conversation with Watching Self: did it help you step back, appraise your ability to cope and generate solutions to problem?
    - Did you feel as though you were losing control?
    - Did you feel negative emotions? What were they? How intense were they?
    - How likely is it that the outcome will be negative after a conversation with your Watching Self?
    - Who is the Watching Self?

Table 3 Typical examples from previous groups

Rule	Rule Break Activating Event	Expected Outcome	What Does Your Watching Self Say?	Desired Outcome
1 Always leave a lot more time than needed	Friend invites for lunch in another town	Daughter won't manage Row when I get back She'll be outside alone	Daughter can look after self Prepare food before I go Speak to her in advance so she knows	All will be OK Will get to see my friend Daughter will be fine

(Continued)

Breaking rules voluntarily

Table 3 (Continued)

Rule	Rule Break Activating Event	Expected Outcome	What Does Your Watching Self Say?	Desired Outcome
2 Do not put self in situations where I appear different from other people; hide my weaknesses	Go to library to ask about taking out talking books	They will say I am not eligible They will think I can't read	Why should it matter what they think? I know I can read Talking books exist because many people take them for many private reasons	I will take out talking books with no problem
3 Don't put self in situations that make demands on memory	Group asks me to buy cake for next week without writing it down; I tell them I might have to write it down as I probably will forget	They make fun of me They laugh at me	We all write to remember; that is what diaries are for; remembering to do something is more important than what you do to remember	I tell them I must write it down to remember and they agree and congratulate me for saying so
4 Hide my weaknesses Hide my emotions	Cook dinner for my boyfriend in front of him	It will go wrong I will burn myself I will burn the food	Would not keep him as boyfriend if he thought me an idiot We have known each other for ages He knows I've had ABI	He will love it Will be a good meal together I will want to do it again Boost my confidence
5 Avoid situations I cannot control Don't risk being made a fool of	Ring up opticians to find out results of eye test to see if I can drive again	Fed up Wonder why I bother Disappointed Won't ever be able drive	If I don't find out I will never drive Whoever rings, result will be same 50/50 chance; worth a try	Passed test Can book driving lesson

4 Next week's assignment and end [15 minutes]

- **Purpose:**
  - Extend participants' range of real-life activities by encouraging them to voluntarily break their dysfunctional and restrictive rules
  - Train in visualising critical events to prepare for in-vivo exposure
  - Improve awareness and co-opting of the Watching Self
  - Train in evolving own solutions to problems

- **Instruction:**
  Please do exercise 2 again but use a different scenario. Remember to use your imagination to visualise the scenario and your conversation with your Watching Self very vividly, as if you were experiencing the whole scene here and now.

Breaking rules voluntarily

- **Reminder:**

  Inform group that next week there will be a virtual reality exposure with relaxation exercise, and it would be useful for participants to bring their recording devices to capture this exercise for playback at home. Participants should also bring pillows to optimise their comfort during relaxation and a scarf with which to cover their eyes to minimise distraction.

Breaking rules voluntarily: confronting our fears, learning to be boss

➤ AIMS AND OVERVIEW

This session is the entry to real-life voluntary rule-break experimentation. It builds on the work of the previous session. It aims to help participants reclaim their sense of self-efficacy by experiencing themselves as being capable of attaining their goals by confronting their fears and managing their anxiety.

The last three sessions have been the scaffolding for trialling voluntary rule breaks and engaging in real-life behavioural experiments with critical events. Relaxation training provides yet another scaffolding level to this end.

Ideally, the training must culminate in participants being able to self-relax in critical situations. Participants ought to so develop the skills to self-relax that when the Watching Self advises them to so do, they can mentally 'chill out' and enter a tranquil state.

Practitioners can use whichever relaxation technique they feel most comfortable with. They may also use a compact disc of their choice.

My preference is **autogenic relaxation**, which uses body awareness and visual imagery. During relaxation, participants lie comfortably on the floor in the group room and cover their eyes with their scarves. The room is prearranged to enable this configuration. I use a stopwatch to time all imagining sequences.

I refrain from giving surreal images, such as waves crashing on the beach or forests with leaves rustling in the wind. Instead, I reinforce a sense of privacy by inviting participants to select a scene of their own choice in which they feel calm, safe and content. I call this image 'your secret/safe place.' I do not ask them to share it with me or with the group. The 'safe place' image complements the feeling of being autonomous in one's own world that the eye-covering scarf generates.

➤ PROCESS NOTES

Objectives and tasks

Objectives: Help participants to

1 **Habituate** to fear-provoking components of critical events
2 **Extinguish** the associations they developed since their ABI between these components and their negative outcome expectations
3 **Develop their own solutions** to problems by co-opting the Watching Self to process the situation
4 **Develop sense of self-efficacy** by experiencing themselves as being capable of attaining their goals by confronting their fears and managing their anxiety

Tasks:

1 Set out this session's purpose and outline [10 minutes]
2 Summarise last week's session and review assignments [15 minutes]

Breaking rules voluntarily: confronting our fears, learning to be boss

3 Explain and describe how to enter a state of relaxation [20 minutes]

4 Help participants select a critical event and relax them as a group for imaginary exposure to the selected critical event [50 minutes]

5 Obtain group feedback on the relaxation exercise [15 minutes]

6 Explain next week's assignment and end the session [20 minutes]

Total time: 130 minutes

1 Welcome and introduction [10 minutes]
As in previous sessions

2 Summary of last session and assignment review [15 minutes]

- **Last session**
  - Automatic thoughts and consequent negative emotions occur primarily when we construe events without evaluating the reality-base of our cognitions, perceptions and interpretations
  - When we construe events 'on-line' in this way, they may engulf us and make us feel that we might lose control
  - We can develop the ability to step back and to reality-test the accuracy of our thoughts and interpretations so as to think through critical events and evolve solutions to the problems they pose

  - We can learn to recognise our Watching Self as the agent that enables us to step back from events and reality-test our cognitions and interpretations
  - By visualising critical events, we learn to call up vivid images of what we need to practise in advance of real-life experiencing

- **Assignment review**
  - **Examples from previous groups:** Table 4 [next page] offers typical examples. It shows that most participants are beginning to achieve positive outcomes. Practitioners reinforce these and use Socratic questioning and guided discovery to attain closure with those who have not done so [Example Assignment 4]. Practitioners also point out that the group shares a great proportion of their rules, anxieties and concerns. Participants explore the reasons for this in a facilitated discussion. Discussions in previous groups have revealed that commonly held negative automatic thoughts and dysfunctional rules reflected the shared loss of self-sameness, continuity and self-efficacy consequent upon the experience of ABI
  - **Present group:** Participants share and discuss the content of both assignments with the group

Breaking rules voluntarily: confronting our fears, learning to be boss

Table 4 Typical assignment results for Session 11

Activating Event	Automatic Thoughts	Rule	Did Your Watching Self Speak? What Did It Say?	Outcome	Emotional Consequence
1 Going to supermarket rather than shop online	I am in people's way People will bump into me and I'll be hurt I won't find what I'm looking for I'll make a fool of myself	Don't put self in situations you can't control Avoid crowds/risk Hide weaknesses	People too busy to judge you personally; they have their own stresses Supermarkets reposition merchandise to sell more goods; no one can be sure of finding what they are looking for. Staff there to help customers; ask them	Got agitated at first but calmed self down	Watching Self did OK
2 Calling DVLA to clarify my driving situation	I won't understand what they say Won't be able to ask for explanation; they will think me a fool	Hide my weaknesses Avoid confrontation so people don't know I am damaged	DVLA call centre will answer; they don't know you personally Many people seek clarification; I did at work before ABI Call centres receive training to explain issues to customers, not to judge them	Kept on imagining and rehearsing; wrote issues down	Went over it with Dad; felt OK
3 Cooking meal without checking with family first if they will like it	I will mess up meal They won't like it They will have to prepare another meal	Check everything before I do anything to make sure I don't make any mistakes Keep harmony; please others	Take something I cook at cookery class to see if they like it Ask if they would like me to bring something from cookery class	Good solution	OK

(Continued)

Breaking rules voluntarily: confronting our fears, learning to be boss

Table 4 (Continued)

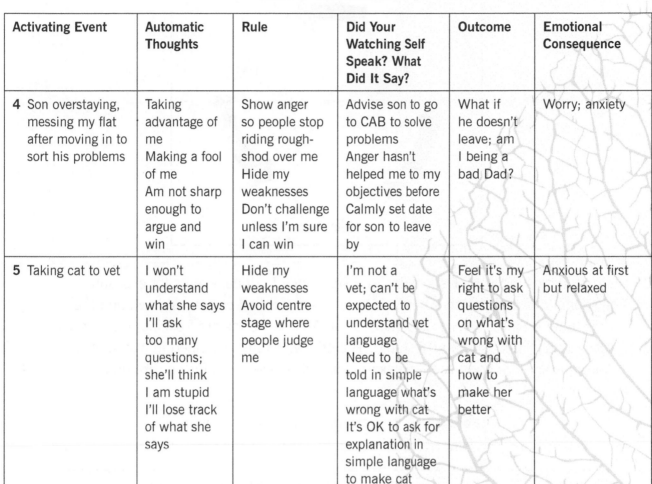

Activating Event	Automatic Thoughts	Rule	Did Your Watching Self Speak? What Did It Say?	Outcome	Emotional Consequence
4 Son overstaying, messing my flat after moving in to sort his problems	Taking advantage of me Making a fool of me Am not sharp enough to argue and win	Show anger so people stop riding rough-shod over me Hide my weaknesses Don't challenge unless I'm sure I can win	Advise son to go to CAB to solve problems Anger hasn't helped me to my objectives before Calmly set date for son to leave by	What if he doesn't leave; am I being a bad Dad?	Worry; anxiety
5 Taking cat to vet	I won't understand what she says I'll ask too many questions; she'll think I am stupid I'll lose track of what she says	Hide my weaknesses Avoid centre stage where people judge me	I'm not a vet; can't be expected to understand vet language Need to be told in simple language what's wrong with cat It's OK to ask for explanation in simple language to make cat better	Feel it's my right to ask questions on what's wrong with cat and how to make her better	Anxious at first but relaxed

3 Learning to enter a state of relaxation [20 minutes]

The key five learning points of relaxation training:

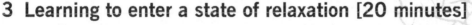

1   Reinforcement mechanism that maintains our dysfunctional rules
    The reinforcement mechanism that maintains negative emotions and action sequences is the sense of relief that occurs when we avoid an anxiety-provoking critical event. The positive emotion we feel upon taking avoidance action increases the likelihood that we will feel negative emotions and take maladaptive action when faced with the same or similar critical event. Our application of our dysfunctional rules, therefore, makes it more likely that we will need to apply them again.

Breaking rules voluntarily: confronting our fears, learning to be boss

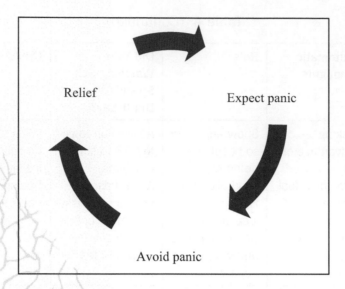

2 Characteristics of SMART scenarios and selection of critical events for exposure

The scenario is a situation where the 'rule' is not applied or breaks down and the dysfunctional core belief is activated. SMART scenarios are Specific, Measurable, Attainable, Realistic and Testable. The critical events described in last session's assignment are good scenario examples. Table 5 sets out further examples of SMART scenarios

Table 5 Further examples of SMART scenarios

Not Smart	Smart
Fear of failure Fear of causing disappointment Fear of causing displeasure	Making a specific mistake on a specific assignment Letting someone down on a specific promise you have made or about a specific expectation they have about you Refusing to carry out a specific request
Fear of losing control Fear of being a burden Fear of being inadequate	A specific instance of involuntary rule break; dropping plate of food on kitchen floor Causing a specific row or disagreement; making a specific mistake Being challenged in a specific situation on a specific issue
Fear of danger	Being in a specific situation perceived as risky; football match, concert

3 Communicating whilst in a relaxed state

Communicating whilst in a relaxed state is done by signalling by hand/finger raising. The relaxed person signals only two mind states: one, when they have got the full and vivid image of the scenario they are visualising; and two, if and when they feel anxiety. Participants must not overlook or minimise the slightest feeling of anxiety but must signal it irrespective of how negligible it may be. There are no other signalling requirements.

Breaking rules voluntarily: confronting our fears, learning to be boss

4   Making relaxation work and developing the skills to self-relax

- Making relaxation work:
  - Imagine only what you have been directed to imagine. Do not embellish, add to or build up your image
  - If you come to the end of your scenario, begin to imagine again and again until you are told to stop thinking about it
  - Make sure to signal clearly; maintain your hand up until I acknowledge your signal
  - Continue imagining yourself in the scenario again and again despite feeling anxious or panicky until told to stop imagining; do not switch off the image
  - If you do not feel anxious, continue to imagine yourself in the scenario; even if you get bored with it, continue to imagine it again and again until told to stop

- Developing the skills to self-relax is a special and effective tool that the Watching Self brings to play in critical situations. The objectives of recording today's relaxation exercise are to
  - Capture this session and practise it regularly to develop skills of self-relaxation
  - Cope effectively with the demands of critical events in day-to-day life by trialling voluntary rule breaks with minimal or no anxiety

4 Imagining that we are experiencing our fear-provoking critical events here and now and allowing ourselves to feel negative emotions [50 minutes]

- **Group room prearranged for relaxation configuration**

- **Acknowledging signals**
  Participants raise hands to signal full access to this image. Practitioners acknowledge the signal with a 'Hmm Hmm' each time a hand is raised.
  All signals are acknowledged in this way.

- **Timing all imaging sequences**[4]
  - Safe place:
    - First safe place image: 5 minutes
    - Subsequent safe place images: 1 to 2 minutes depending on anxiety levels
    - No image interval between safe place and next image; 60 seconds
  - Imaginary exposure to critical event; exposure duration depends on groups' signalled anxiety level
    - No anxiety signalled: first exposure: 3 minutes; second exposure: up to 6 minutes
    - Anxiety signalled: participants continue to imagine until told to stop. First anxiety exposure ends after 2 minutes. Event reimagined in next three exposures up to 7 minutes. In between each anxiety image, participants return to safe place and imagine that for 2 minutes

- **Ending relaxation**
  Following the last exposure, participants return to safe place and stay there for 2 minutes. They are then instructed 'stop imagining' for a 'no image' relaxation period of 1 minute.
  At the end of this practitioners say, 'now I will count up to 5 slowly, and then please remove your scarves and open your eyes.' Count up to 5 at the rate of 3 seconds per number.

Breaking rules voluntarily: confronting our fears, learning to be boss

5 Feedback [20 minutes]

- **Quality of participants' relaxation and imagery**
  - Were imagined scenarios vivid?
  - What were the accompanying emotions?
  - Were they easy to manage?

- **Watching Self**
  - Did Watching Self help manage negative emotions effectively?
  - Did Watching Self offer constructive solutions to the problems posed by critical events?

- **Safe place**
  - Was retreat to safe place relaxing? Helpful?

6 Next week's assignment and end [10 minutes]

Three assignments:

1 **Rehearsal:** Practise this session's recorded relaxation exercise in full as recorded at least three times during the week

2 **Behavioural experiment:** Trial the imagined critical event in real-life at least three times during the week
3 **Recording:** Record the outcome in the assignment table in the handout

Practitioners:

- Link next weeks' assignment to participants' feedback of the exercise
- Facilitate expression of any concerns about the behavioural experiments and alleviate them
- Remind participants to bring recording devices, pillows and scarves for next week's relaxation exercise

Are our negative beliefs about ourselves true?

➤ AIMS AND OVERVIEW

This session prepares participants to build self-efficacy. Self-efficacy refers to people's beliefs in their ability to exercise influence over the events that affect their lives by producing requisite levels of performance to attain their goals.[5]

The session's key aim is to reconfigure participants' experience of themselves as agents that possess the potential to attain their goals and to master the critical demands that impact their day-to-day lives. Their work with the Watching Self and behavioural experiments has gone some way towards achieving this aim by making it easier for participants to dislodge some of their negative core beliefs about themselves.

➤ PROCESS NOTES

Objectives and tasks

Objectives:

1 Extend participants' sense of mastery over critical events
2 Help participants construe effective coping as mastery of critical events
3 Prepare participants to evaluate core beliefs

Tasks:

1 Set out this session's purpose and outline [5 minutes]
2 Summarise last week's session and review assignments [20 minutes]
3 Extend participants' mastery of a new set of critical events by running a relaxation/imaginary exposure exercise [50 minutes]

4 Obtain group feedback on the relaxation exercise [20 minutes]
5 Facilitate a discussion on evaluating core beliefs to answer the question: Are our negative beliefs about ourselves true? [25 minutes]
6 Explain next week's assignment and end the session [10 minutes]

Total time: 130 minutes

1 Welcome and introduction [5 minutes]

As in previous sessions

2 Summary of last session and assignment review [20 minutes]

- **Last session**
  - The five key points of relaxation:
    1 Reinforcement mechanism that maintains our dysfunctional rules
    2 Characteristics of SMART scenarios and selection of critical events for exposure
    3 Communicating whilst in a relaxed state
    4 Making relaxation work
    5 Developing the skills to self-relax
  - Experience of relaxation and imaginary exposure to critical events

- **Assignment review**
  - **Examples from previous groups:** Table 6 on the next page sets out typical assignment results. They show that most participants achieve positive outcomes in their behavioural experiments
  - **Present group:** Participants share and discuss the content of both assignments with the group

Are our negative beliefs about ourselves true?

○ **Discussion Points**

♦ Reinforce achievements reported in assignment results by pointing out that success with behavioural experiments represents mastery of challenges, which participants had been avoiding until now

♦ Reinforce participants' ability to stick with assignments and to attain goals

♦ Use Socratic questioning and guided discovery to attain closure with participants who have not obtained positive outcomes with behavioural experiments

♦ Link assignment results with the relaxation exercise of the next section: Participants who have achieved positive results in their behavioural experiments extend their mastery by trialling new critical events. Participants who have obtained equivocal results may choose to trial last week's scenario or select a new one

Table 6 Typical assignment results from previous groups

Critical Event Scenario	Violated Rule	Automatic Thoughts	What Did I Feel During Behavioural Experiment?	How Did My Watching Self Help Me Manage the Situation?	Outcome	What Did I Feel at End of Behavioural Experiment?
Went to visit Mother on a school day	Don't do anything that might cause row with daughter Don't put self in situations you can't control	Will be late getting back Traffic will be bad Bus will not arrive Will be pushing for time	Anxious	Tell daughter in advance; prepare everything; she will cope	Got to see Mum	Satisfaction
Cooked dinner for my boyfriend in front of him	Hide my weaknesses Hide my emotions	It will be crap It will not be good enough I will look an idiot I will be useless Will not cope I will burn myself I will burn the food	Anxious	You've cooked before; you know how to cook Make a simple meal Not a sin to ask him to help	He loved it Was a good meal I will do it again	Boosted my confidence Very good

(Continued)

Are our negative beliefs about ourselves true?

Table 6 (Continued)

Critical Event Scenario	Violated Rule	Automatic Thoughts	What Did I Feel During Behavioural Experiment?	How Did My Watching Self Help Me Manage the Situation?	Outcome	What Did I Feel at End of Behavioural Experiment?
Rang Spec savers to find out the results of my eye test to see if I can drive again	Avoid situations I cannot control	I won't have passed I don't know what to say	Anxious	Result won't change by asking You discuss more difficult things every week in the group	I rang and I have passed	Pleased with self
Made bread at cookery class and took it home to family	Check everything before you do anything	They won't like it They will laugh at me They will bin it	Anxious	If the class liked it, no reason why family should not like it If they don't like it ask them how they would prefer it You don't like all food put in front of you	They liked it a lot	Very pleased

3 Relaxation/imaginary exposure to a new set of critical events [50 minutes]

- Reminder of the key five learning points of relaxation training
- Relaxation exercise [as in previous session]

4 Group feedback [20 minutes]

Comparison of this session's imaginary exposure with that of the last session and that of their home-rehearsal in terms of:

- Quality of participants' relaxation and imagery
  - Were imagined scenarios vivid?
  - What were the accompanying emotions?

- Watching Self
  - Did Watching Self help manage negative emotions effectively?
  - Did Watching Self offer constructive solutions to the problems posed by critical events?

- Safe place
  - Was retreat to safe place relaxing? Helpful?

Are our negative beliefs about ourselves true?

5 Are our negative beliefs about ourselves true? group discussion [25 minutes]

The purpose of this discussion is to help participants doubt the veracity of their dysfunctional self-appraisals by

- **Recalling negative core beliefs:** Practitioners draw a table on the board; ask participants to select one negative core belief
- **Identifying the evidence for and against** within the context of their achievements in the last four group sessions [sessions 10 to current; Table 7 sets out examples from previous groups]; ratings are recorded on board
- **Discussion points:** Reality-testing of ratings with use of guided discovery and Socratic questioning; draw attention to the role of the Watching Self in countering the evidence for the negative beliefs

Table 7 Typical examples from previous groups of rating evidence for and against negative core beliefs about self

Negative Core Belief 1		Negative Core Belief 2	
I Am Incompetent		I Am a Burden	
Evidence For	Evidence Against	Evidence For	Evidence Against
1 I mess up everything	1 Didn't mess up meal I cooked	1 I don't go to work and others look after me	1 Have insurance; structure my time and help with home and kids
2 I can't get anything right	2 Dealt with daughter OK, visited Mum OK	2 I am physically disabled	2 Am independent with my aids
3 I forget everything	3 Can remember with lists like everybody else	3 I make mistakes and make it harder for everyone else	3 Everyone makes mistakes; I am aware of and correct my mistakes; being at home to help with chores makes life easier for family
4	4	4	4

6 Next week's assignment and end [10 minutes]
Four assignments:

1 **Rehearsal:** Practise this session's recorded relaxation exercise in full as recorded at least three times during the week

Are our negative beliefs about ourselves true?

2 **Behavioural experiment:** Trial the imagined critical event in real-life at least three times during the week

3 **Recording[6]:** Record outcome in the assignment table in the handout

4 **Evaluating negative core beliefs:** Participants select two negative core beliefs, identify their components and rate the evidence for them and against them in light of their achievements in the last four sessions

Evidence for our beliefs and our rules

➤ AIMS AND OVERVIEW

The aim of this session is to restructure the negative beliefs participants have developed about their capabilities, autonomy and self-worth in consequence of their ABI.

The session highlights that next week is the programme's last session. It congratulates the group on its achievements in extending the frontiers of its mastery over critical demands and encourages participants to trial a wider range of critical events during the coming week.

Experience with previous groups shows that this session sometimes brings forth safety behaviours or understanding difficulties during evaluation of core beliefs and rules. This manifests in participants describing the symptoms rather than the impact of ABI consequences on their sense of self. In such cases, practitioners gently explore the changes that have occurred in participants' self-perceptions to enable them to return to the fold of the group. This work occurs within the context of the group. If practitioners feel that they are not getting through, then they bring their guided discovery to a close.

Previous group discussions of evaluations of negative core beliefs reveal that the belief most resistant to change is *'I am not safe.'*[7] One way of dealing with this is to attempt to alter the anticipation of the probability of risk with reference to accident statistics: risk of car accidents is significantly higher than that of plane crashes, for example.[8]

➤ PROCESS NOTES

Objectives and tasks

Objectives:

1 Instil the idea that participants can exercise control over situations they perceive as threatening by extending their mastery over a wider range of critical events

2 Demonstrate that they are able to attain their goals by helping them to incorporate their recent achievements within their post-ABI belief and rule systems

Tasks:

1 Set out this session's purpose and outline [5 minutes]
2 Summary of last session and assignment review [20 minutes]
3 Group discussion on assignment results in the context of goal attainment [30 minutes]
4 Group exercise: Rating the consequences of a dysfunctional post-ABI life rule [35 minutes]
5 Next week's assignment and end [20 minutes]

Total time: 110 minutes

1 Welcome and introduction [5 minutes]

As in previous sessions

Evidence for our beliefs and our rules

2 Summary of last session and assignment review [20 minutes]

- **Last session:**
  - Repeated relaxation exercise with imaginary exposure to critical events
  - Identified the evidence for and against our negative core beliefs

- **Assignment review:**
  - **Examples from previous groups:**
    - ◆ **Relaxation/imaginary exposure rehearsal and behaviour experiment** positive outcomes included:
      - ✧ Went shopping with shopping list
      - ✧ Took cat to vet
      - ✧ Telephoned DVLA
      - ✧ Booked yoga class
      - ✧ Made apple crumble and jam tarts at cookery class, took home without first asking for permission
  - **Evaluating negative core beliefs:** Table 8 presents sample evaluations.

Table 8 Sample core belief evaluations

Negative Core Belief 01: I Am Not Safe		Negative Core Belief 02 I Am Faulty Goods	
Evidence For	**Evidence Against**	**Evidence For**	**Evidence Against**
1 Memory poor	1 Am still in one piece	1 Am physically dependent	1 Am almost independent with my aids
2 Get tired quickly	2 House still standing	2 Can't find my words when I speak	2 Can still hold my own in conversation
3 Mobility poor	3 Not afraid to ask for help	3 Get tired quickly	3 I know what tasks I can and can't do; preserve my energy
4 Can't see well	4 Have people who look out for me	4 My friends no longer visit me	4 Some do; I now know who my real friends are
5 Have been mugged	5 More aware of risk now; can protect self	5 Can't multi-task as I used to	5 Am coping with the multiple frame-breaking changes of ABI Have intelligence to learn new ways of doing things
6 Had fits in supermarket before	6 I have not had a fit for years, am on anticonvulsants Have been assessed as fit to drive	6	6

(Continued)

Evidence for our beliefs and our rules

Table 8 (Continued)

Negative Core Belief 3 Can't Rely On Self		Negative Core Belief 4 I Am Weak	
7 Make mistakes	**7** I know when I make them and correct them	**7** Afraid to challenge people	**7** Spoke to DVLA, asked shop for discount; asked shop to explain directions for use of new gadget
8 Can't make decisions	**8** Have made several important decisions recently: took on voluntary work. Sold my car, took my dog to training class, helped my neighbour	**8** Can't tell friends about my worries and difficulties since ABI	**8** Told friends and family about feeling unsafe and worries about crowded places
9 Can't solve problems as well as before	**9** I can solve them if I come back to them later; I have learned to look at them differently, but it takes longer	**9** I keep away from people because I worry they will think there is something wrong with me	**9** Booked yoga class, went to party, went to library
10 Memory poor	**10** I can remember OK with memory aids	**10** Afraid of people in authority	**10** Asked Dad to explain letter from DVLA

- **Present group:** Participants share and discuss the content of both assignments with the group. Practitioners congratulate participants on the successful outcomes of their behavioural experiments and the quality of their evaluation of their core beliefs.

3 Group discussion: revisiting assignment results in the context of goal attainment [30 minutes][9]

- **Objective:** demonstrate that participants are already:
  - Exercising control over an increasing range of critical events
  - Setting and attaining an increasing range of goals

- **Discussion:**
  - Participants name the goals and outcomes of their behavioural experiments within the framework of pre-drawn shared goal table on board
  - Practitioners help sort these goals into categories
  - Participants:
    + Share examples of related specific behaviour experiments
    + Share with the group their ability to engage in these activities before the programme and what they felt before, during and after the behavioural experiment
    + Name their negative core beliefs and receive help in grouping together those held in common
    + Identify and evaluate shared core beliefs
    + Explore how belief changes have come about

- ◆ If belief change has not occurred, practitioners elicit reasons with the use of Socratic questioning and guided discovery
- ○ Tables 9 and 10 offer sample goal and belief examples from previous groups.

Table 9 Behavioural experiment goal and achievement table [sample shared goals]

Shared Goal	Shared Achievement Yes/No	Was I Able To Engage in These Activites Before the Group Programme?
Be comfortable in crowded places		
Be comfortable on telephone with strangers		
Stop avoiding people		
Be comfortable with perceived authority		
Use post-ABI aids without being ashamed		
Undertake difficult tasks in the presence of other people		

Table 10 Shared negative core belief evaluation table [sample shared beliefs]

Shared Belief	Belief Is Not True of Me Now [Indicate With X]	Belief Is Still True of Me [Indicate With X]
I am faulty goods		
I am not safe		
I am weak		
I am not in control		
I am worthless		
I am incompetent		

4 Group exercise: rating the consequences of our life rules [35 minutes]

- **Objective:** for participants to realise that as their self-concept alters and leads to changes in their core beliefs, their life rules become obsolete and even disadvantageous.
- **Process:** participants select a shared life rule which practitioners note on flip chart. A facilitated group discussion follows within the framework of the table
- **Discussion** explores:
  - ○ Recollections of critical events in which participants relied on this rule
  - ○ Critical events in which the rule broke unexpectedly
  - ○ What were the consequences?
  - ○ Was this rule ever effective?
  - ○ Table 11 offers a sample rule from previous groups

Table 11 Analysing the consequences of a commonly held sample life rule

Life Rule	Negative Consequences of Adhering to Rule	Positive Consequences of Rule Break	Should We Maintain This Rule?
If I can please others all the time they will not criticise me	• Belittles self, you feel you are not worthy • Lack of faith in self • Lack of self-worth • No confidence in own judgment • Degraded • No confidence to say no • Takes away your identity • Lose respect from others • Others are not grateful and take you for granted.	• Empowerment • Giving back your self-worth • Restoring identity • No self-resentment • No anger at self • Gain respect for self • Gain respect from others • People will not put on you • Will not take advantage of you	No; it belittles you; raises your anxiety [can't please everyone all the time]

5 Next week's assignment and end [20 minutes]
Four assignments:

1 **Rehearsal:** Practise recorded relaxation exercise in full with a new set of critical event scenarios
2 **Behavioural experiment:** Trial the imagined new critical event in real-life at least three times during the week
3 **Recording:** Record behavioural experiment outcome in the assignment table in the handout
4 **Evaluating Dysfunctional Life Rules:** Select two dysfunctional life rules and identify the negative consequences of adhering to them and the positive consequences of breaking them

Goodbye: ABI – a life-long learning experience

➤ AIMS AND OVERVIEW

This is the last session of this programme. Its aim is to enable participants to consolidate and enduringly retain the learning gains they have achieved throughout the programme.

➤ PROCESS NOTES

Objectives and tasks

Objectives:

To inspire participants to transcend the adverse cognitive, behavioural, emotional and interpersonal consequences of ABI by

1 Developing acknowledgment and acceptance of post-ABI changes
2 Reclaiming the locus of control over their capabilities, over their functioning and over events that affect their lives
3 Gaining mastery over their post-ABI life order
4 Building belief in self-efficacy through recognition and acknowledgment of their achievements

Tasks:

1 Set out this session's purpose and outline [5 minutes]
2 Summarise last week's session and review assignments [20 minutes]
3 Encourage participants to conduct real-life behavioural experiments with a new set of critical events [10 minutes]
4 Identify the key learning points of the programme's three modules [30 minutes]
5 Facilitate a group discussion on recognising self-efficacy in ourselves [35 minutes]

6 Say goodbye and end the session: Reframe ABI experience as one of life-long learning [20 minutes]

Total time: 120 minutes

1 Welcome and introduction [5 minutes]

As set out in task list

2 Summary of last session and assignment review[10] [20 minutes]

- **Last session**
  - Reviewed assignments in the context of attaining goals
  - Rated the consequences of dysfunctional life rules
  - Recalled and articulated material that they learned during the previous session

- **Assignment review**
  - **Examples from previous groups:**
    - ♦ **Relaxation/imaginary exposure rehearsal and behaviour experiment:** Examples of achievements with new critical events include:
      - ✧ Enrolled in adult college of further education
      - ✧ Joined gym
      - ✧ Went to voluntary work interview
      - ✧ Enrolled in cane training
      - ✧ Enrolled in NVQ course
    - ♦ **Evaluating dysfunctional life rules:** Table 12 sets out two examples of rule evaluation
  - **Present group:** Participants share and discuss the content of both assignments with the group

Goodbye: ABI – a life-long learning experience

○ **Discussion:**

♦ Congratulating successful outcomes of behavioural experiments and quality of evaluation of dysfunctional life rules

♦ Exploring reasons for maintaining dysfunctional rules and beliefs

♦ Highlighting that these belief rule systems are inherently self-limiting and actually lead to feeling and becoming helpless in the various arenas of day-to-day life

Table 12 Sample dysfunctional life rule evaluation

Life Rule	Negative Consequences of Adhering to Rule	Positive Consequences of Rule Break	Should We Maintain This Rule?
1 If I hide my weaknesses, people will not know I am useless/incompetent	• Reinforces belief 'I am crap' • Gives me low self-worth • Reduces your identity • Deskills you • Reduces self-expression • Reinforces lucky escape but you then start worrying again about next time.	• Gain confidence • You win the challenge and increase self-esteem • Increases your coping ability	No; it belittles you; raises your anxiety in long run; stops you from dealing with adversity
2 If I avoid confrontation, people won't realise I am useless/damaged	• Allows people to take advantage of me • Makes me lose self-respect • People think I am a pushover • I end up losing anyway	• I obtain what I am entitled to • People respect me • I respect myself • I learn not be ashamed of my impairments	No; it makes you ashamed of your ABI; you can never come to terms with it; it makes you a loser

3 Life-long practice of relaxation/imaginary exposure to new sets of perceived threats followed by behavioural experiments [10 minutes]

Practitioners invite participants to practise relaxation and engage in behavioural experiments in the face of perceived threats on a life-long basis. This is a coping tool which they have acquired and should make use of whenever critical events demand it.

4 Identifying the key learning points of the programme's three modules: group discussion [30 minutes]

• **Objective:** for participants to highlight, acknowledge and commit to retaining and to using the material that they feel has helped them most.

• **Process:**

○ Participants contribute learning points for each module and these are noted on flip chart

Goodbye: ABI – a life-long learning experience

○ Reference to discussion of learned helplessness [discussion in present group assignment review, Section 3] during recall of Module 2 learning points [discussion in present group assignment review, Section 3, page 94, Discussion bullet point 3]
○ Examples of participants' actions that have exerted an influence on their environment
  • **Examples from previous groups:** Table 13

Table 13 Sample key learning points of programme modules

Modules	What Did We Do?	What Did We Learn?	Key Learning Points
1 Recognising change	We analysed ourselves to see if we are different from the way we were before ABI	ABI had changed us. Changes were uncomfortable; not easy to come to terms with them. The most important change was that most of us were extrovert before ABI and had become introvert after ABI	1 ABI had changed us 2 We denied/ignored/tried to hide these changes from ourselves and from others 3 We 'took it lying down'
2 Exploring change	Because of these changes, our core beliefs became dysfunctional and needed to be addressed	We saw ourselves in a very bad light, as stupid, worthless and incompetent. We set up life rules and protective behaviours to hide these. So really we kind of stopped functioning; stopped living.	4 Denying and hiding changes made us: • unable to cope • lose control • feel helpless
3 Mastering change	We learned tools such as relaxation and behavioural experiments to face our problems and start living again	We learned to relax and chill out, not to get anxious. We learned to push boundaries with behavioural experiments to break the rules and the behaviours. We learned to deal with things when they go wrong instead of beating ourselves up about them.	5 Come to terms with, accept and learn to master changes resulting from ABI 6 Cope with stressful problems 7 Set and attain our goals 8 Push our boundaries 9 We are competent in what we undertake

5 Recognising self-efficacy in ourselves: group discussion [35 minutes]

• **Focus:** group decision on whether or not it recognises efficacy in its recent as well as lifetime endeavours as a unit and as individuals. Table 14 gives examples from my groups.
• **Process:** Participants give examples of efficacy and these are noted on flip chart.
• **Discussion:**
  ○ Key learning points of Module 3 demonstrate participants' ability to attain its goals and to accomplish tasks
  ○ Participants give further examples of self-efficacy
  ○ Exploring how these rich examples of lifetime self-efficacy have been cancelled out by the adverse consequences of ABI

Goodbye: ABI – a life-long learning experience

- ◆ Insidious slide into learned helplessness
- ◆ Inability to share the frame-breaking emotional, cognitive and behavioural changes
- ○ Participants identify Module 3 learning points that demonstrate emergence from learned helplessness

- **Examples from previous groups:**

Table 14 Do we believe we are effective? Samples from my groups

Key Learning Points From Module 3	Examples of Recent Self-Efficacy	Examples of Lifetime Self-Efficacy
• Come to terms with and learn to accept changes resulting from ABI	Learned how to write again Did a presentation using notes Enrolled in cane-training course Told friend I worried about my safety after ABI Asked friend to speak slowly	
• Cope with stressful problems	Stayed calm when friend shouted at me because I was late Passed driving test Managing well in crowds on my own Gave boyfriend birthday party Advocated for and stood by daughter Did well at voluntary work interview Tackled difficult computer situation well	Managed to have a child despite the risks Went through stressful divorce Gave up smoking Helped friend through crisis
• Attain goals	Passed my apprenticeship exam Told I was a model tenant Praised by tutor at class Got hold of talking books	Bought first house Brought up children to be polite Wife agreed to marry me – still married after 20 years Got promoted at work Held down sales job
• Push our boundaries	Agreed to fundraise for charity Enrolled in NVQ course Completed gym course Went away for weekend Joined dog-training class Organised friend's market stall	Always there for the children Brought up children well; people comment on it Completed further education diploma Took control and organised cousin's wedding Went travelling

6 Goodbye: ABI – a life-long learning experience [20 minutes]

- **Discussion:**
  - ○ Participants describe how they felt and feel about their ABI experience pre- and post-group: post-group descriptions identify the positive changes that have come about

because of their achievements both in and outside of the group programme. Any positive change does not detract in any way from the adverse and painful characteristics of ABI

  ○ Both sets of descriptions noted on flip chart
- **Examples from previous groups:** Table 15

Table 15 Sample of pre- and post-group descriptions of ABI experience

Pre-Group Description of ABI Experience	Post-Group Positive Changes In Me Brought About by ABI
• 'Why me?'	• Wiser and stronger
• Catastrophe	• More chilled out about problems
• Terrible	• Better able to put things in context – wiser
• Frightening	• More aware of mistakes and correcting them
• Enraging	• Better at monitoring self; more self-aware
	• Better at finding new ways of dealing with problems
	• Better able to understand people's suffering
	• More compassionate with self
	• Now more motivated to actively strive to adapt to life post-ABI
	• Now more motivated to improve; more actively involved in rehabilitation

- **Goodbye:** ABI is such a momentous, frame-breaking experience that it remains a life-long benchmark against which to measure almost all of life's other critical incidents. By comparison with ABI, most of the scenarios which participants imagined and trialled in behaviour experiments during the course of the programme pale into utter insignificance.

This perhaps is the key learning point of the programme.

Notes
1 Cicerone and Azulay (2007)
2 In Participants' Handout
3 In Participants' Handout
4 Time lines reflect general rules and may vary according to the group and the discretion of the practitioner.
5 Bandura (1977)
6 Both tables in Participants' Handout
7 This is consistent with research on threat appraisals; see Riley et al. (2010).
8 According to Amoros et al. (2006), in France, in the 1997–2001 period, there were 59,714 car accident casualties. Belcastro and Foster (2010) report in the 1999–2008 period, there were 1,991 airplane crash fatalities.
9 Present group's exercise Tables 2, 3 and 4 are put on the board in advance of the session.
10 Tables 1, 2, 3 and 4 for present group pre-drawn on flip chart.

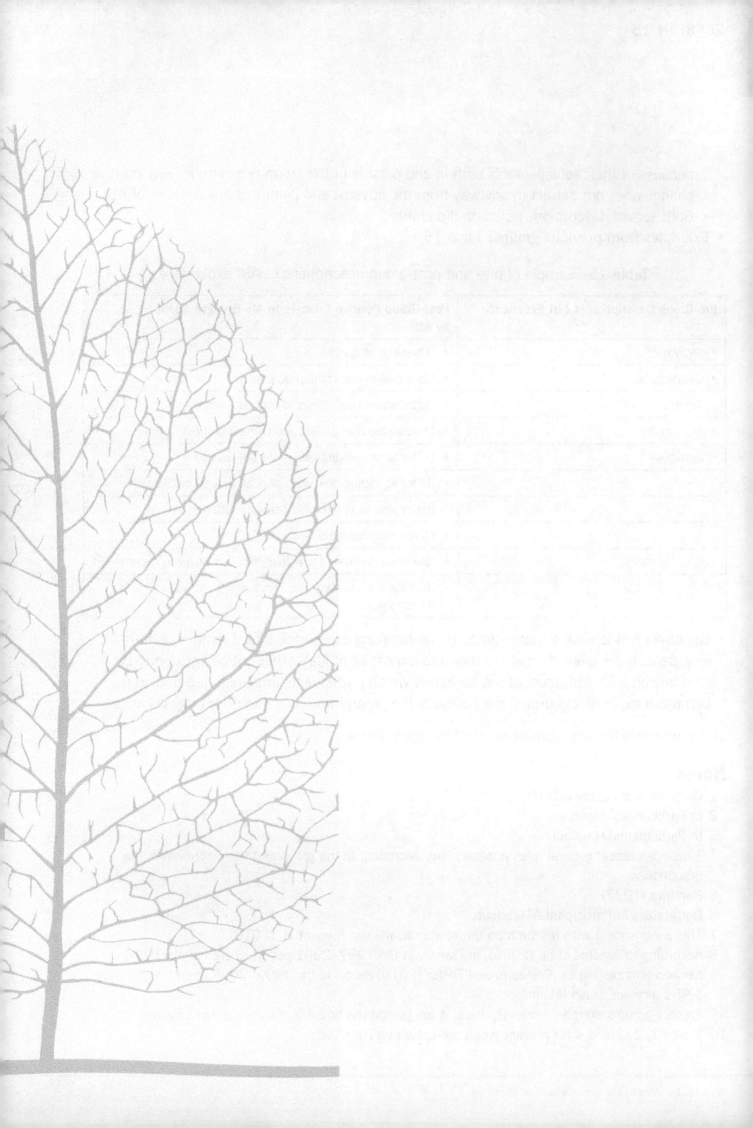

PARTICIPANTS' HANDOUT

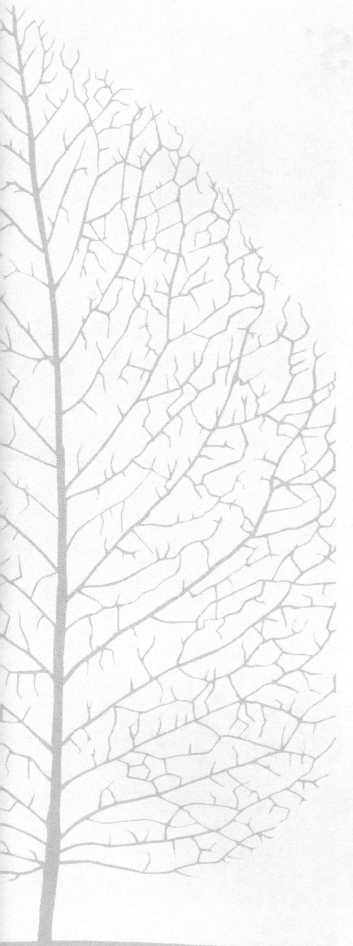

MODULE 1

Recognising change

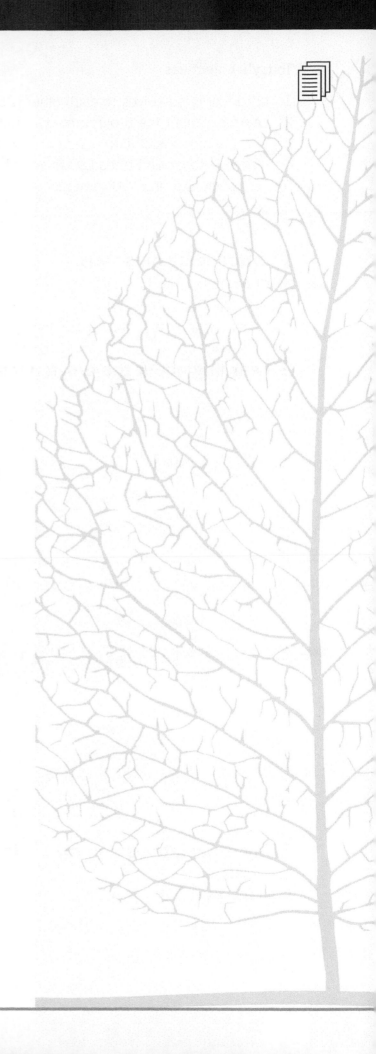

Today's objectives

1 Introducing ourselves to each other [25 minutes]
2 Learning about the programme [15 minutes]
3 Sharing our expectations and our anxieties [40 minutes]
4 Agreeing to ground rules [20 minutes]
5 Feedback and end [20 minutes]

Total time: 120 minutes

1 Introducing ourselves

- My name
- My brain injury: how, when?
- My life: what was it like before my injury; what is it like now?

2 Learning about the programme

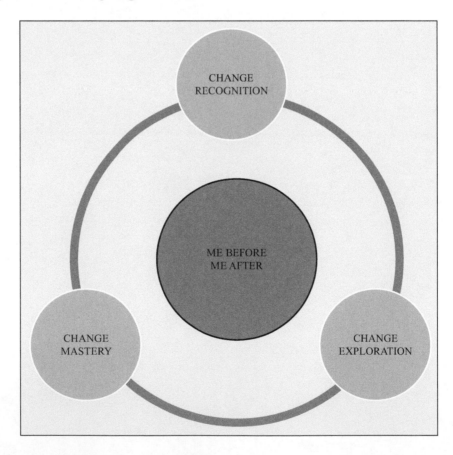

3 My expectations and my anxieties

My expectations
My anxieties

Welcome

4 Agreeing ground rules

1 Commitment
This is your programme. Commit to it.

2 Respect
Listen actively – respect others when they are talking. The goal is not to agree – it is to gain a deeper understanding of ourselves and of each other.

3 Alcohol and other drugs
Group members cannot participate in the group under the influence of alcohol or other mind-altering drugs.

4 Exclusive relationships
Dating and other exclusive relationships between or among group members are not allowed.

5 Attendance
You must attend every meeting unless an emergency arises.

6 Confidentiality
Anything said between any two or more group members at any time is part of the group and is confidential. The single exception to this rule of confidentiality applies to the group leader. If the group leader believes that someone is in danger, the leader has a professional obligation to take direct action in order to keep everyone safe.

7 Assignments
You must complete all your assignments.

8 Tell me if you are unhappy
I can't help you if I don't know! Together we can work things out.

5 My feedback and end

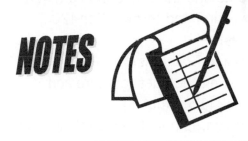

How do I make relationships? extroversion vs. introversion

Welcome and introduction [15 minutes]

- Log books
- Handouts

Session objectives
1. Identify any differences in the way we make relationships now and how we made them before ABI
2. Explore the reasons for these differences
3. Identify what we want to change about ourselves after ABI

Session outline
1. Welcome and Introduction [15 mins]
2. Extroversion and Introversion [20 minutes]
3. Discussion [20 mins]
4. Completing the questionnaire and feedback [15 minutes]
5. Discussion: Is how I make relationships now different from how I made them before my brain injury? [30 minutes]
6. Next week's assignment and end [15 minutes]

                    Total time: 115 minutes

1 Extroversion and introversion [30 minutes]
Making relationships: Extrovert or Introvert?

Extrovert people are sociable, outgoing and have many friends. They take the initiative in making new friends; they like meeting new people and can be the life and soul of the party. They like to be involved in many groups and activities, welcome change, make quick decisions and don't like to be alone.

Introvert people are deep thinkers who have to consider the ins and outs of situations before they make decisions. They have few but close friends. They tend to prefer to be alone and involve themselves in solitary activities. They prefer reading to meeting people. They do not like change and can work alone for long periods.

2 Discussion [20 mins]

3 Completing the questionnaire [15 minutes]

4 Questionnaire feedback and discussion: is how I make relationships now different from how I made them before my brain injury? [30 minutes]

EXTROVERT/INTROVERT: Please complete this questionnaire by putting a cross beside the item that describes you best for both **AFTER** and **BEFORE** your ABI. Please answer every question. When you finish, add up your crosses in each column. Work out also the grand total of your crosses and put them in the appropriate columns at the end of the continuation table.

How do I make relationships? extroversion vs. introversion

Extroversion [E]	After ABI	Before ABI	Introversion [I]	After ABI	Before ABI
	X	X		X	X
1 I like getting my energy from taking active part in what is going on around me			1 I like getting my energy from dealing with what is inside my own head: my own ideas, memories, images, and reactions that are in my inner world		
2 I like it when there are lots of people around me			2 I often prefer doing things alone or with one or two people I feel comfortable with		
3 I like taking action and making things happen			3 I take time to think things through so that I have a clear idea of what I'll be doing when I decide to act		
4 I generally feel part of the world around me and feel at home in it			4 I feel most comfortable and 'at home' in my own company or in the company of one or two people that I know well		
5 I often understand a problem better when I can talk out loud about it and hear what others have to say			5 I feel comfortable solving my problems on my own		
6 I am a 'people person'			6 I am 'reserved' and tend to keep myself to myself		
TOTAL					

How do I make relationships? extroversion vs. introversion

Extroversion [E]	After ABI	Before ABI	Introversion [I]	After ABI	Before ABI
	X	X		X	X
7 I feel comfortable in groups of people and like doing things in them			**7** I feel comfortable being alone and like things I can do on my own		
8 I have a wide range of friends and know lots of people			**8** I prefer to know just a few people well		
9 I sometimes jump too quickly into an activity and don't allow enough time to think it over			**9** I sometimes spend too much time thinking things through and don't move into action quickly enough		
10 Before I start a project, I sometimes forget to stop and get clear on what I want to do and why			**10** I sometimes forget to check with the outside world to see if my ideas really fit the experience		
11 I would change the world if I could			**11** I would understand the world if I could		
TOTAL					
GRAND TOTAL					

Our group scores

Participant	Now: After ABI		Then: Before ABI	
	Extrovert	Introvert	Extrovert	Introvert
me				

How do I make relationships? extroversion vs. introversion

5 Next week's assignment and end [15 minutes]

Assignment 1: EXTROVERT/INTROVERT: Please complete the Exercise questionnaire (Assignment Table 1) by putting a cross beside the item that describes you best for both **AFTER** and **BEFORE** your ABI. Please answer every question. When you finish, add up your crosses in each column. Work out also the grand total of your crosses and put them in the appropriate columns at the end of the continuation table.

Assignment 2: HOW HAVE I CHANGED? Please summarise the ways in which you have changed in your own words: the way you see yourself now, after your brain injury, compared with the way you saw yourself then, before your brain injury. I have given three examples to get you started.

Assignment 3: Based on Tables 1 and 2, please identify and list the changes you want to make about yourself after your ABI.

Assignment: EXTROVERT/INTROVERT: Please complete this questionnaire by putting a cross beside the item that describes you best for both **AFTER** and **BEFORE** your ABI. Please answer every question. When you finish, add up your crosses in each column. Work out also the grand total of your crosses and put them in the appropriate columns at the end of the continuation table.

Table 1

Extroversion [E]	After ABI	Before ABI	Introversion [I]	After ABI	Before ABI
	X	X		X	X
1 I feel comfortable in groups of people and like doing things in them			1 I feel comfortable being alone and like things I can do on my own		
2 I have a wide range of friends and know lots of people			2 I prefer to know just a few people well		
3 I sometimes jump too quickly into an activity and don't allow enough time to think it over			3 I sometimes spend too much time thinking things through and don't move into action quickly enough		
TOTAL					

(Continued)

How do I make relationships? extroversion vs. introversion

Table 1 (Continued)

Extroversion [E]	After ABI	Before ABI	Introversion [I]	After ABI	Before ABI
	X	X		X	X
4 Before I start a project, I sometimes forget to stop and get clear on what I want to do and why			**4** I sometimes forget to check with the outside world to see if my ideas really fit the experience		
5 I would change the world if I could			**5** I would understand the world if I could		
6 I like getting my energy from taking active part in what is going on around me			**6** I like getting my energy from dealing with what is inside my own head: my own ideas, my own memories, images, and my reactions that are in my inner world		
7 I like it when there are lots of people around me			**7** I often prefer doing things alone or with one or two people I feel comfortable with		
8 I like taking action and making things happen			**8** I take time to think things through so that I have a clear idea of what I'll be doing when I decide to act		
TOTAL					

(Continued)

How do I make relationships? extroversion vs. introversion

Table 1 (Continued)

Extroversion [E]	After ABI	Before ABI	Introversion [I]	After ABI	Before ABI
	X	X		X	X
9 I generally feel part of the world around me and feel at home in it			**9** I feel most comfortable and 'at home' in my own company or in the company of one or two people that I know well.		
10 I often understand a problem better when I can talk out loud about it and hear what others have to say			**10** I feel comfortable solving my problems on my own.		
11 I am a 'people person.'			**11** I am 'reserved' and tend to keep myself to myself		
TOTAL					
GRAND TOTAL					

Table 2 HOW HAVE I CHANGED? Please summarise the ways in which you have changed in your own words: the way you see yourself now, after your brain injury, compared with the way you saw yourself then, before your brain injury. I have given three examples to get you started.

Me Before My ABI	Me After My ABI
More busy	Less confident
More friends	Think more
Thought less about things	Speak less

SESSION 2
How do I make relationships?
extroversion vs. introversion

Table 3 Based on Tables 1 and 2, please identify and list the changes you want to make about yourself after your ABI.

What Do I Want to Change About Myself After My ABI?
1
2
3
4
5
6
7
8
9
10

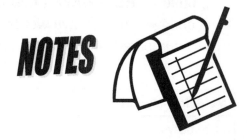

How do I gather information?
sensing vs. intuition

Welcome and introduction
[10 minutes]

Today's objectives

1 Identify any differences in the way we gather information after and before ABI
2 Explore the reasons for these differences
3 Identify what we would like to change about ourselves after ABI

Session Outline

1 Summary of last session and assignment review [20 mins]
2 How I gather information: sensing and intuition [40 minutes]
3 Exercise: which type are you? [15 minutes]
4 Discussion: Is how I gather information now different from how I did before my brain injury? [30 minutes]
5 Next week's assignment and end [15 minutes]

1 Summary of last session and assignment review [20 minutes]

2 How I gather information: sensing and intuition [40 minutes]

Sensing and intuition are the information-gathering functions. They describe how we collect, understand and process information.

Examples of information you gathered during the past week.

1
2
3
4

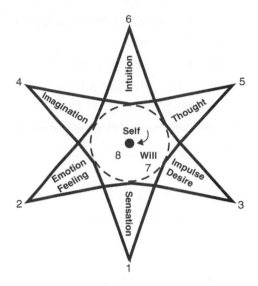

People who prefer sensing trust information that is in the present, tangible, and concrete: that is, information that can be understood by the five senses. They tend to distrust hunches, which seem to come 'out of nowhere.' They prefer to look for details and facts. For them, the meaning is in the here and now and in the facts.

People who prefer intuition trust information that is less dependent upon the senses. They are more interested in future possibilities. For them, the meaning is in the underlying pattern that goes beyond the facts.

Sensing types pay attention to physical reality: what they see, hear, touch, taste and smell. They are concerned with what is actual, present, current and real. They notice facts and remember details that are important to them. They are good with their hands, and like to get on with the task at hand. They are not interested in what might happen in the future or what might be possible.

How do I gather information? sensing vs. intuition

 They do not think of **what might happen tomorrow or next week if . . .** They look at **what is actually happening now**. When they try to solve a problem, they just look at the options that are relevant now; they don't bother to think about what might happen in the future.

Intuitive types pay attention to impressions or to the meaning and patterns of the information they get. They prefer to learn by thinking a problem through than by hands-on experience. They are interested in new things and what might be possible.

They think more about the future than the past. They remember events more as an impression of what it was like than as actual facts or details of what happened

They concentrate on the future and on possibilities. They are always thinking **what might happen if . . .** They are less interested in what is going on in the here and now. They are imaginative and have many 'gut feels.' When they solve a problem, they look at many more options than might be necessary.

3 Exercise: which type are you? [15 minutes]

Completing the questionnaire and feedback

Do you pay more attention to information that comes in through your five senses **(Sensing)**, or do you pay more attention to the patterns and possibilities that you see in the information you receive **(Intuition)**? Put a cross on the statement that applies to you best.

How do I gather information?
sensing vs. intuition

SENSING/INTUITION: Please complete this questionnaire by putting a cross beside the item that describes you best for both **AFTER** and **BEFORE** your ABI. Please answer every question. When you finish, add up your crosses in each column. Work out also the grand total of your crosses and put them in the appropriate columns at the end of the continuation table.

Sensing [S]	After ABI	Before ABI	Intuition [N]	After ABI	Before ABI
	X	X		X	X
1 I remember events as a series of photographs of what actually happened			1 I remember events by what I read 'between the lines' about their meaning		
2 I pay attention to physical reality			2 I am interested in doing things that are new and different		
3 I look at the facts to solve a problem			3 I like to see the big picture before I settle down to thinking about the facts		
4 I am a here-and-now person; I just concentrate on what is happening now			4 I trust impressions, symbols, and gut-feel more than what I actually experience through my senses		
5 I start with what is here now; I am not interested in what might happen later			5 I solve problems by thinking through possible solutions rather than by trying them out		
6 I trust experience and actions; I am not interested in words and symbols			6 I am a future-oriented person; not a here-and-now person		
TOTAL					

Sensing [S]	Before ABI	After ABI	Intuition [N]	Before ABI	After ABI
7 When I have a problem, I look at the options that are present now; I am not interested in what options may present in the future.			**7** I concentrate on what might happen rather than on what is.		
8 Sometimes I pay so much attention to facts that I miss possibilities.			**8** I prefer the theoretical to the practical		
9 I value things that are useful			**9** I am imaginative and have many gut-feels		
10 I learn best by doing things rather than by reading about them			**10** When I solve a problem, I consider many more options than are necessary because I want to make sure that I have not missed anything that might go wrong in the future.		
11 When I have a problem, I look at the options that are present now; I am not interested in what options may present in the future.			**11** I trust my impressions about things rather than my senses		
12 Sometimes I pay so much attention to facts that I miss possibilities.			**12** I concentrate on what might happen rather than on what is.		
13 I make decisions based on what my senses tell me here and now; I do not take any notice of my impressions			**13** I value things that are beautiful and meaningful; their usefulness is not important		
TOTAL					
GRAND TOTAL					

4 Discussion: Is how I gather information now different from how I did before my brain injury? [30 minutes]

5 Next week's assignment and end

Assignment: **SENSING/INTUITION:** Please complete this questionnaire by putting a cross beside the item that describes you best for both **AFTER** and **BEFORE** your ABI. Please answer every question. When you finish, add up your crosses in each column. Work out also the grand total of your crosses and put them in the appropriate columns at the end of the continuation table.

Table 4

Sensing [S]	After ABI	Before ABI	Intuition [N]	After ABI	Before ABI
	X	X		X	X
1 I remember events as a series of photographs of what actually happened			1 I remember events by what I read 'between the lines' about their meaning		
2 I pay attention to physical reality			2 I am interested in doing things that are new and different		
3 I look at the facts to solve a problem			3 I like to see the big picture before I settle down to thinking about the facts		
4 I am a here-and-now person; I just concentrate on what is happening now			4 I trust impressions, symbols, and gut-feel more than what I actually experience through my senses		
5 I start with what is here now; I am not interested in what might happen later			5 I solve problems by thinking through possible solutions rather than by trying them out		
6 I trust experience and actions; I am not interested in words and symbols			6 I am a future-oriented person; not a here-and-now person		
TOTAL					

(Continued)

How do I gather information? sensing vs. intuition

Table 4 (Continued)

Sensing [S]	Before ABI	After ABI	Intuition [N]	Before ABI	After ABI
	X	X		X	X
7 When I have a problem, I look at the options that are present now; I am not interested in what options may present in the future			7 I concentrate on what might happen rather than on what is		
8 Sometimes I pay so much attention to facts that I miss possibilities			8 I prefer the theoretical to the practical		
9 I value things that are useful			9 I am imaginative and have many gut-feels		
10 I learn best by doing things rather than by reading about them			10 When I solve a problem, I consider many more options than are necessary because I want to make sure that I have not missed anything that might go wrong in the future		
11 When I have a problem, I look at the options that are present now; I am not interested in what options may present in the future			11 I trust my impressions about things rather than my senses		
12 Sometimes I pay so much attention to facts that I miss possibilities			12 I concentrate on what might happen rather than on what is		
13 I make decisions based on what my senses tell me here and now; I do not take any notice of my impressions			13 I value things that are beautiful and meaningful; their usefulness is not important		
TOTAL					
GRAND TOTAL					

Table 5 HOW HAVE I CHANGED? Please summarise the ways in which you have changed in your own words: the way you see yourself now, after your brain injury, compared with the way you saw yourself then, before your brain injury. I have given three examples to get you started.

Me Before My ABI	Me After My ABI
I was more interested in the future	Less motivated for information
Used my intuition as much as I used my senses	Rely on my senses more to make sure I am right
I had more confidence in the way I did things	Can't trust my senses any more

Table 6 WHAT CHANGES DO I WANT TO MAKE Based on Tables 4 and 5, please identify and list the changes you want to make about yourself after your ABI.

What Do I Want to Change About Myself After My ABI?
1
2
3
4
5
6
7
8
9
10

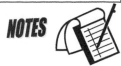

NOTES

How do I make decisions? thinking vs. feeling

Welcome and introduction [10 minutes]

Today's objectives

1 Identify any differences in the way we make decisions now after ABI and how we made them before ABI
2 Explore the reasons for these differences
3 Identify what we would like to change about ourselves after ABI

Session outline

1 Summary of last session and assignment review [20 minutes]
2 How we make decisions: **Thinking** and **Feeling** [40 minutes]
3 Completing the questionnaire and feedback [15 minutes]
4 Discussion: is how I make decisions now different from how I did before my brain injury [30 minutes]
5 Next week's assignment and end [10 minutes]

Total time: 115 minutes

1 Summary of last session and assignment review [20 minutes]

2 How we make decisions: thinking and feeling [40 minutes]

A '**Thinker**' makes decisions in a rational, logical, impartial manner, based on what they believe to be fair and correct by pre-defined rules of behaviour.

A '**Feeler**' makes decisions on the individual case, in a subjective manner, based on what they believe to be right within their own value systems. For example, say you are a nurse, a doctor, a fire fighter. Your organisation imposes a pay cut on you that you think is unjust. Would you go on strike, even though you know that the public depends on your services, or would you carry on working?

When someone makes a decision that is based on logic and reason, they are operating in **Thinking** mode. When someone makes a decision that is based on their value system, or what they believe to be right, they are operating in **Feeling** mode. We all use both modes for making decisions, but we put more trust into one mode or the other.

Thinking people analyse the given facts and arrive at a decision through a logical thinking process. They tend to make decisions quite quickly and are not interested in how people will be affected by their decisions. They can make quite tough decisions, such as sacking people, for example. They focus on making the best decision that will be the best solution to the problem at hand. They are not interested in the moral implications of such decisions or if people's feelings will be hurt by the consequences of their decision.

Feeling-focused people are people-oriented and concerned with the moral implications of their decisions. They focus on the feelings of the people that will be affected by their decision. They are concerned that their decisions uphold the principles of justice, fairness and morality. Because of this, feeling-focused people tend to take a long time to make decisions. They want to make sure that their decision does not violate a moral principle in which they have a strong belief.

How do I make decisions?
thinking vs. feeling

Decisions that we find most difficult are those in which we **have conflicts** between our **Thinking** and **Feeling** sides. In these situations, our dominant preference will take over. Decisions which we find easy to make and feel good about are usually a result of our feeling and thinking sides being in synchrony.

3 Completing the questionnaire and feedback [15 minutes]

THINKING/FEELING: Please complete this questionnaire by putting a cross beside the item that describes you best for both **AFTER** and **BEFORE** your ABI. Please answer every question. When you finish, add up your crosses in each column. Work out also the grand total of your crosses and put them in the appropriate columns at the end of the continuation table.

Thinking [T]	After ABI	Before ABI	Feeling [F]	After ABI	Before ABI
	X	X		X	X
1 I make decisions quite quickly because I want to solve the problem as quickly as possible without spending too much time on how this will impact the people concerned			1 I take a long time to make decisions because I want to make sure that my decision does not violate any moral principles and upsets the people concerned as little as possible		
2 I make decisions in a rational, logical, impartial manner, based on what I believe to be fair and correct by pre-defined rules of behaviour			2 I make decisions on the individual case, in a subjective manner based on what I believe to be right within my own value system		
3 I am a solution-oriented person and make decisions by analysing the given facts. I focus on making the best decision that will be the best solution to the problem at hand. I am not interested in the moral implications of such decisions or			3 I am a people-oriented person and take care to make sure that the implications of my decisions do not violate the moral principles in which I believe		

(Continued)

How do I make decisions?
thinking vs. feeling

Thinking [T]	After ABI	Before ABI	Feeling [F]	After ABI	Before ABI
	X	X		X	X
if people's feelings will be hurt by its consequences					
4 When I make decisions I like to rely on facts and impersonal information irrespective of how it will affect the people concerned			4 When I make decisions, I like to think of how it will affect the people concerned and how they are likely to feel		
5 When I make decisions, I like to be impersonal; I do not let my personal wishes or other people's wishes influence me			5 When I make decisions, I take into account what people care about and take account of the viewpoints of the people involved in the situation		
6 I like to make decisions on technical and factual matters where I can use my logic			6 I like to make decisions in matters where it is important to establish what is best for people and where I can rely on the principles of what is right and what is wrong		
7 I believe that telling the truth is more important than being tactful about people's feelings			7 When I make decisions, I like to make sure that I maintain harmony between people		
8 When I make decisions I sometimes ignore or do not value the 'people' aspect of the situation			8 I believe that being tactful about people's feelings is more important than telling the 'cold truth'		
9 I look for logical solutions or explanations to everything			9 I look for what is important to others and express concern for others		

(Continued)

How do I make decisions?
thinking vs. feeling

Thinking [T]	After ABI	Before ABI	Feeling [F]	After ABI	Before ABI
	X	X		X	X
10 I make decisions with my head and want to be fair			10 I make decisions with my heart and want to be compassionate		
11 Others sometimes see me as too task-focused and uncaring or indifferent			11 Others sometimes see me as too idealistic, soft or indirect		
TOTAL					
GRAND TOTAL					

4 Discussion: is how I make decisions now after my brain injury different from how I did before my brain injury [30 minutes]

5 Next week's assignment and end [10 minutes]

Assignment: THINKING/FEELING: Please complete this questionnaire by putting a cross beside the item that describes you best for both **AFTER** and **BEFORE** your ABI. Please answer every question. When you finish, add up your crosses in each column. Work out also the grand total of your crosses and put them in the appropriate columns at the end of the continuation table.

Table 7

Thinking [T]	Now	Pre-ABI	Feeling [F]	Now	Pre-ABI
	X	X		X	X
1 I make decisions quite quickly because I am concerned to solve the problem as quickly as possible without spending too much time on how this will impact the people concerned			1 I take a long time to make decisions because I want to make sure that my decision does not violate any moral principles and upsets the people concerned as little as possible		

(Continued)

Table 7 (Continued)

Thinking [T]	Now	Pre-ABI	Feeling [F]	Now	Pre-ABI
	X	X		X	X
2 I make decisions in a rational, logical, impartial manner, based on what I believe to be fair and correct by pre-defined rules of behaviour			**2** I make decisions on the individual case, in a subjective manner based on what I believe to be right within my own value system		
3 I am a solution-oriented person and make decisions by analysing the given facts. I focus on making the best decision that will be the best solution to the problem at hand. I am not interested in the moral implications of such decisions or if people's feelings will be hurt by its consequences			**3** I am a people-oriented person and take care to make sure that the implications of my decisions do not violate moral principles in which I believe		
4 When I make decisions I like to rely on facts and impersonal information irrespective of how it will affect the people concerned			**4** When I make decisions, I like to think of how it will affect the people concerned and how they are likely to feel		
5 When I make decisions, I like to be impersonal; I do not let my personal wishes or other people's wishes influence me			**5** When I make decisions, I take into account what people care about and take account of the viewpoints of the people involved in the situation		

(Continued)

How do I make decisions?
thinking vs. feeling

Table 7 (Continued)

Thinking [T]	Now	Pre-ABI	Feeling [F]	Now	Pre-ABI
	X	X		X	X
6 I like to make decisions on technical and factual matters where I can use my logic			6 I like to make decisions in matters where it is important to establish what is best for people and where I can rely on the principles of what is right and what is wrong		
7 I believe that telling the truth is more important than being tactful about people's feelings			7 When I make decisions, I like to make sure that I maintain harmony between people		
8 When I make decisions I sometimes ignore or do not value the 'people' aspect of the situation			8 I believe that being tactful about people's feelings is more important than telling the 'cold truth'		
9 I look for logical solutions or explanations to everything			9 I look for what is important to others and express concern for others		
10 I make decisions with my head and want to be fair			10 I make decisions with my heart and want to be compassionate		
11 Others sometimes see me as too task-focused and uncaring or indifferent			11 Others sometimes see me as too idealistic, soft or indirect		
TOTAL					
GRAND TOTAL					

How do I make decisions? thinking vs. feeling

Table 8 HOW HAVE I CHANGED? Please summarise the ways in which you have changed in your own words: the way you see yourself now, after your brain injury compared with the way you saw yourself then, before your brain injury. I have given three examples to get you started.

Me Before My ABI	Me After My ABI
I didn't used to worry about what people thought	Can't rely on feelings any more
I used my feelings as much as I used my thinking	I am more concerned about the consequences of my actions now
I had more confidence in my decisions	Can't trust my thinking any more

Table 9 WHAT CHANGES DO I WANT TO MAKE? Based on Tables 1 and 2, please identify and list the changes you want to make about yourself after your ABI.

What Do I Want to Change About Myself After My ABI?
1
2
3
4
5
6
7
8
9

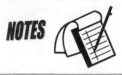

NOTES

How do I organise my life?
judging vs. perceiving

Welcome and introduction [10 mins]

Today's objectives

1 Identify any differences in the way we organise our lives after and before ABI
2 Explore the reasons for these differences
3 Identify what we would like to change about the way we organise our lives after ABI

Session outline

1 Summary of last session and assignment review [20 minutes]
2 How I organise my life: **Judging** and **Perceiving**: [30 minutes]
3 Completing the questionnaire and feedback [15 minutes]
4 Discussion: is how I organise my life now different from how I did before my brain injury? [30 minutes]
5 Next week's assignment and end [15 minutes]

Total time: 120 minutes

1 Summary of last session and assignment review [20 minutes]

2 How I organise my life: judging and perceiving [30 minutes]

Judging people like to plan for everything and do not like the unexpected to be sprung upon them. Their holidays are arranged well in advance, their appointments are set in advance and they are extremely punctual. They are highly organised and highly

efficient. They do not like to change their programme or plans to fit in with something new and they certainly do not like last-minute changes.

Perceiving people are rather disorganised although they know where everything is. Their desks are full of papers that require attention, and their rooms tend to be in need of putting in order. They do not like to commit to advance plans and consider the unexpected as a welcome challenge. They are easily adaptable and like to learn new ways of doing things. They tend not to keep time or appointments well because they easily attend to something new that has come their way. They tend not to plan their holidays or anything in advance and thrive on chaos.

Judgers approach life in a structured way, creating plans and organizing their world to achieve their goals and desired results in a predictable way. They like to take charge of their environment and to make choices early. They are self-disciplined and decisive, and like to make decisions quickly and get the job done.

Perceivers look upon structure as being limiting. They prefer to keep their choices open so they can cope with the many problems that life will put in their way. They are curious and like to expand their knowledge. They are tolerant of other people's differences and will adapt to fit into whatever the situation requires. They tend to avoid or put off decisions and instead prefer to explore problems and situations.

How do I organise my life? judging vs. perceiving

3 Completing the questionnaire and feedback [15 minutes]

JUDGING/PERCEIVING: Please complete this questionnaire by putting a cross beside the item that describes you best for both **AFTER** and **BEFORE** your ABI. Please answer every question. When you finish, add up your crosses in each column. Work out also the grand total of your crosses and put them in the appropriate columns at the end of the continuation table.

Judging [J]	After ABI	Before ABI	Perceiving [P]	After ABI	Before ABI
	X	X		X	X
1 I prefer a planned, orderly way of life			1 I prefer a flexible, spontaneous way of life		
2 I like to have things settled and organised			2 I like to understand the world rather than to organise it		
3 I like to bring life under control as much as possible			3 I am always open to new experiences and to new ways of doing things		
4 I like to have things decided			4 I tend to decide what to do as I do it rather than make a plan in advance		
5 I like to know what the task is and get on with it			5 I am loose and casual; I don't like to plan things in advance		
6 I like to make lists of things to do			6 I don't like to separate work and play; I like to mix them		
7 I like to get my work done before playing			7 I work in bursts of energy		
8 I avoid deadlines by planning my work well in advance			8 I am stimulated by an approaching deadline so I never plan my work		
9 Sometimes I focus so much on making the decision that I miss new information			9 I like the unexpected and look upon it as a welcome challenge		
10 I don't like unexpected things to be sprung upon me			10 I am not very punctual because I get sidetracked by new things that come my way		
TOTAL					

(Continued)

How do I organise my life?
judging vs. perceiving

Judging [J]	After ABI	Before ABI	Perceiving [P]	After ABI	Before ABI
	X	X		X	X
11 I don't like last-minute changes			11 My house is generally in a mess but I like it that way		
12 I make sure my house is always in good order			12 Sometimes I stay open to new information too long, and I miss making important decisions		
13 I schedule things well in advance			13 I postpone making decisions because I want to see what other options are available		
14 I like to make a decision about an issue quickly so that I can move on			14 I like to do things at the last minute		
15 Others see ne as well organised but not always flexible			15 Others see me as disorganised but I know where everything is		
16 I am always punctual and structured			16 I don't like to commit to plans too far in advance		
TOTAL					
GRAND TOTAL					

4 Discussion: is how I organise my life now after my brain injury different from how I did before my brain injury [30 minutes]

5 Next week's assignment [15 minutes]

- **Tasks:**
  - **Assignment 1:**
    - Complete the questionnaire
    - Add up your scores
    - Are your ratings any different from those you made during the session?
  - **Assignment 2:** describe in your own words how and why you have changed
  - **Assignment 3:** go through your session log and record your Pre- and post-ABI preferences on all four dimensions together with your pre- and post-ABI ratings
  - **Assignment 4:** record the first letter of each of your four pre- and post-ABI preferences and give a short summary of how you have changed on all four of them
  - **Assignment 5:** Identify the preferences which you wish to change back to the way they were pre-ABI

How do I organise my life?
judging vs. perceiving

 ASSIGNMENT 1: Please complete this questionnaire by putting a cross beside the item that describes you best for both **AFTER** and **BEFORE** your ABI. Please answer every question. When you finish, add up your crosses in each column. Work out also the grand total of your crosses and put them in the appropriate columns at the end of the continuation table.

Judging [J]	After ABI	Before ABI	Perceiving [P]	After ABI	Before ABI
	X	X		X	X
1 I prefer a planned, orderly way of life			1 I prefer a flexible, spontaneous way of life		
2 I like to have things settled and organised			2 I like to understand the world rather than to organise it		
3 I like to bring life under control as much as possible			3 I am always open to new experiences and to new ways of doing things		
4. I like to have things decided			4 I tend to decide what to do as I do it rather than make a plan in advance		
5 I like to know what the task is and get on with it			5 I am loose and casual; I don't like to plan things in advance		
6 I like to make lists of things to do			6 I don't like to separate work and play; I like to mix them		
7 I like to get my work done before playing			7 I work in bursts of energy		
8 I avoid deadlines by planning my work well in advance			8 I am stimulated by an approaching deadline so I never plan my work		
9 Sometimes I focus so much on making the decision that I miss new information			9 I like the unexpected and look upon it as a welcome challenge		

(Continued)

ASSIGNMENT 1 (Continued)

Judging [J]	After ABI	Before ABI	Perceiving [P]	After ABI	Before ABI
	X	X		X	X
10 I don't like unexpected things to be sprung upon me			**10** I am not very punctual because I get sidetracked by new things that come my way		
11 I don't like last-minute changes			**11** My house is generally in a mess but I like it that way		
12 I make sure my house is always in good order			**12** Sometimes I stay open to new information too long, and I miss making important decisions		
13 I schedule things well in advance			**13** I postpone making decisions because I want to see what other options are available		
14 I like to make a decision about an issue quickly so that I can move on			**14** I like to do things at the last minute		
15 Others see ne as well organised but not always flexible			**15** Others see me as disorganised but I know where everything is		
16 I am always punctual and structured			**16** I don't like to commit to plans too far in advance		
TOTAL					
GRAND TOTAL					

How do I organise my life?
judging vs. perceiving

ASSIGNMENT 2: HOW MY LIFESTYLE HAS CHANGED Please summarise the ways in which you have changed in your own words: the way you see yourself now, after your brain injury, compared with the way you saw yourself then, before your brain injury. I have given three examples to get you started.

Me After My ABI	Me Before My ABI
I need to know what will happen next	I enjoyed last minute arrangements
I leave things to take care of themselves	I liked to take charge of things
I don't like sudden change	I never planned my weekends and holidays

ASSIGNMENT 3: Go through your notes across all four group sessions and record your post-ABI and pre-ABI preferences with your scores in the table below.

	Post-ABI [NOW]	Pre-ABI [THEN]
	Score	Score
EXTROVERSION [E]		
INTROVERSION [I]		
SENSING [S]		
INTUITION [N]		
THINKING [T]		
FEELING [F]		
JUDGING [J]		
PERCEIVING [P]		

How do I organise my life?
judging vs. perceiving

ASSIGNMENT 4: Record the first letter of each preference for both post-ABI and pre-ABI in the table below. Give a short description of how you have changed.

Me Before ABI	Me After ABI	Short Description Of How I Have Changed	Which Preference Do I Wish To Change?

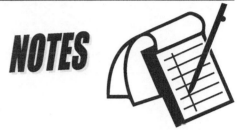

MODULE 2

Exploring change

How we think impacts how we behave

Welcome and introduction [10 minutes]

Today's objectives

1 Develop understanding of the link between our thinking and our feelings
2 Develop understanding of the link between our thinking and our behaviour
3 Develop our ability to become aware of the negative consequences of the way we think

Session outline

1 Summary of last session and assignment review [20 minutes]
2 How my thinking impacts how I feel and how I behave [30 minutes]
3 Exercise: identifying the outcomes of my thinking [20 minutes]
4 Discussion: what are the outcomes of my thinking? [30 minutes]
5 Next week's assignment and end [15 minutes]

Total time: 125 minutes

1 Summary and assignment review [20 minutes]

2 How what I think impacts how I feel and how I behave [30 minutes]

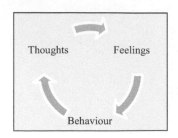

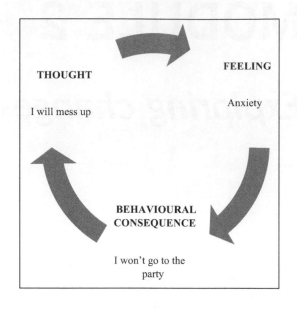

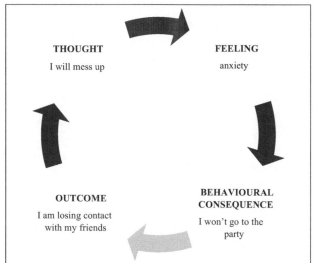

3 Exercise: Identifying the outcomes of my thinking [20 minutes]

Complete the table by giving examples of three of your thoughts in the **THOUGHT** column; stating how each makes you feel in the **FEELING** column; and how you behave as a result of each in the **BEHAVIOURAL CONSEQUENCES** column. Then state the outcome of your thoughts on your lifestyle in the **OUTCOME** column. Exercise Table 1 gives two examples to get you started.

Thought	Feeling	Behavioural Consequences	Outcome
I will mess up	Anxiety	Don't go to the party	Don't meet my friends; don't make new friends
There might be a stampede at the football match	Anxiety	Don't go to football matches any more	Don't go to venues that my friends go to; lose contact with my friends

4 Discussion: What are the emotional and life-quality outcomes of my negative thinking? [30 minutes]

5 Next week's assignment and end [15 minutes]

How we think impacts
how we behave

 ASSIGNMENT 1: Please complete the table by giving examples of at least five of your thoughts in the **THOUGHT** column; stating how each makes you feel in the **FEELING** column; and how you behave as a result of each in the **BEHAVIOURAL CONSEQUENCE** column.

Thought	Feeling	Behavioural Consequence
1	1	1
2	2	2
3	3	3
4	4	4
5	5	5
6	6	6
7	7	7
8	8	8
9	9	9
10	10	10
TOTAL		

ASSIGNMENT 2: THE OUTCOMES OF MY THOUGHT-FEELING-BEHAVIOUR CYCLES: Please describe the outcomes of each of your five thoughts. Are these outcomes positive or negative? How do they make you feel? Complete the table by stating your thoughts in the **THOUGHT** column, its emotional consequence in the **FEELING** column, whether their outcomes are positive or negative in the +/− column, and how these outcomes make you feel in the **EMOTION** column. The table offers two examples.

Thought	Feeling	Behavioural Consequence	Outcome	+/−	Emotion: How Do I Feel About This Outcome?
I will mess up	Anxiety	I don't go to parties any more	I don't meet my friends; I don't make new friends	−	Isolated/alone
There might be a stampede at the football match	Anxiety	I don't go to football matches any more	I don't go to crowded venues that my friends go to; I lose contact with friends	−	Isolated/cut off

How we think impacts how we behave

ASSIGNMENT 3: Do you wish to change the outcomes of your Thought-Feeling-Behaviour Cycles? How? Please complete the table.

Outcome	Do I Wish to Change This Outcome? Yes/No	How?
I don't meet new people	Yes	Not to worry about what people think
I don't go to crowded venues that my friends go to	Yes	Not to worry about safety issues
1		
2		
3		
4		
5		
6		
7		
8		
9		

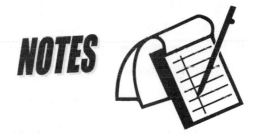

NOTES

How we think impacts how we behave: automatic thoughts before/after ABI

Welcome and introduction [10 minutes]

Today's objectives

1 Develop understanding of automatic thoughts
2 Explore the automatic thoughts we have developed since our ABI
3 Realise the core beliefs which generate them

Session outline

1 Summary of last session and assignment review [20 minutes]
2 My automatic thoughts after/before ABI [30 minutes]
3 Exercise: my automatic thoughts after/before ABI [20 minutes]
4 Discussion: the core beliefs which generate my post-ABI automatic thoughts [30 minutes]
5 Next week's assignment and end [15 minutes]

Total time: 125 minutes

1 Summary and assignment review [20 minutes]

2 My automatic thoughts before/after ABI [30 minutes]

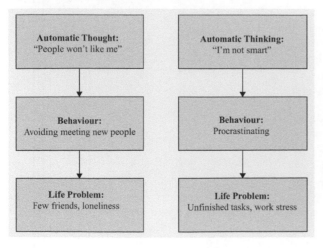

Automatic thoughts are thoughts or visual images that we may not be aware of unless we focus our attention on them. They are part of a habitual pattern of thinking. We think of them as **factual representations of reality**. We believe they are true, so we do not assess their validity.

Automatic thoughts

- Are transient
- Are short and specific
- Occur extremely rapidly before, during or immediately after the event
- Occur in the stream of consciousness
- Do not occur in sentences but may consist of a few key words or images
- Do not arise from careful thought
- Do not occur in a logical series of steps such as problem solving
- Happen involuntarily

Activating events

The events that activate our automatic thoughts are **Activating** or **Critical Events**. These events trigger our negative automatic thoughts and feelings.
Automatic thoughts derive from our past experience. Your ABI experience in its entirety is a **critical, activating event**.

How we think impacts how we behave: automatic thoughts before/after ABI

3 Exercise: my automatic thoughts before/after ABI [20 minutes]

Please complete the table by selecting an activating event which you have experienced both before and after your ABI. It could be going to a concert or football match, helping the children with their homework, cooking a family meal, or an argument. Identify your immediate automatic thoughts and the feelings that they produced both after and before your ABI. Rate these feelings, both after and before your ABI, from 0 to 5 for their negative quality such as anxiety, depression and anger. A rating of 0 indicates no negative emotion; a rating of 5 indicates maximum negative emotion.

After ABI			Before ABI		
Activating Event	Automatic Thought	Feeling Rate From 1 To 5 0 = No Negative Emotion; 5 = Maximum Negative Emotion	Same/Similar Activating Event; Recalled Or Imagined	Automatic Thought	Feeling Rate From 1 To 5 0 = No Negative Emotion; 5 = Maximum Negative Emotion

4 Discussion: The core beliefs which generate my post-ABI automatic thoughts [30 minutes]

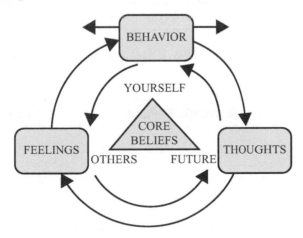

We remember our experiences and store them in our minds as memories. They are our mental stores of **core beliefs**.

We construct core beliefs about ourselves, others and the world. These serve as filters for ongoing experience, allowing us to come to conclusions about events automatically.

How we think impacts how we behave: automatic thoughts before/after ABI

Your ABI experience in its entirety is a **critical, activating event**. It would have created both a set of new automatic thoughts and reinforced some old negative ones as a result of your accumulating post-ABI life experience. Now, post-ABI, each time an activating event faces you, it will stimulate your **mental store of core beliefs**. You will interpret and judge the activating event in terms of core your beliefs.

5 Next week's assignment and end [15 minutes]

1 Please complete the table by selecting three activating events which you have experienced both AFTER and BEFORE your ABI. Identify the immediate automatic thoughts and the feelings that this event produced both AFTER and BEFORE your ABI. Rate these feelings from 0 to 5 for their negative quality. A rating of 0 indicates no negative emotion; a rating of 5 indicates maximum negative emotion.

After ABI			Before ABI		
Activating Event	Automatic Thought	Feeling Rate From 1 To 5 0 = No Negative Emotion; 5 = Maximum Negative Emotion	Same/Similar Activating Event; Recalled Or Imagined	Automatic Thought	Feeling Rate From 1 To 5 0 = No Negative Emotion; 5 = Maximum Negative Emotion
1					
2					
3					

2 Please identify the core beliefs underlying the three activating events you have listed in Assignment Table 1.

Activating Event	Automatic Thought	Core Belief
1		
2		
3		

3 Please make a list of your post-ABI core beliefs.

My Post-ABI Core Belief List
1
2
3
4
5

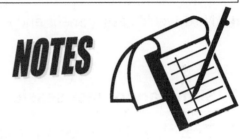

NOTES

How we manage our negative core beliefs: rules and protective behaviours

 Welcome and introduction [10 minutes]

Today's objectives

Explore how we manage our negative core beliefs:

1 Conditional beliefs or rules
2 Protective behaviours

Session outline

1 Summary of last session and assignment review [20 minutes]
2 Exercise: how we manage our negative core beliefs [35 minutes]
3 Discussion: conditional behaviours or rules and protective behaviours [30 minutes]
4 Next week's assignment and end [15 minutes]

Total time: 110 minutes

1 Summary of last session and assignment review [20 minutes]

2 Exercise: How we manage our negative core beliefs [35 minutes]

Please complete the table by selecting an actual activating event. Identify the immediate automatic thought and its underlying core belief. Then describe what you actually did.

Activating Event	Automatic Thought	Core Belief	Behavioural Consequence

3 Discussion: conditional beliefs or rules and protective behaviours [30 minutes]

- **Conditional Beliefs/Rules**

    It is unusual for a person who has a core belief that they are flawed to think that they are 'flawed' *all the time* because such people usually have memories which conflict with this belief.

    For example, we do not feel worthless or incompetent when a family member or friend shows us appreciation of what we have done for them, or when we have worked hard at a task and completed it perfectly.

How we manage our negative core beliefs: rules and protective behaviours

We therefore develop **conditional beliefs**, or **rules**, which we think of as 'if-then' statements. They are conditional, because we do not know that they are true; we assume they are true. For example, if we feel good about ourselves when a family member expresses appreciation of our help, we might develop a rule that reads, *'If people show me appreciation, then I might be okay,'* or *'If people don't show me any appreciation, then I am worthless.'*
If we feel good about ourselves when we complete a task perfectly, then we are likely to develop a rule that reads something like, *'If I am successful at everything I do, I might not be incompetent,'* or *'If I am not totally successful at everything I do, then I'm incompetent.'*
These rules ensure that we behave in certain ways so as to keep the negative belief 'I am worthless' or 'I am incompetent' away from our immediate awareness. They force us to behave in certain ways. For example, we feel obliged to overwork at tasks to produce perfect performance or to always please people, to feel competent or good about ourselves.

- **Protective Behaviours**
  This framework of core beliefs and rules is supported by certain **protective** or **safety behaviours**. These protective behaviours protect us from the activation of negative core beliefs. An example of a safety behaviour is when we behave in ways which lead others to show us their appreciation of what we have done. The appreciation we seek and receive enables us to avoid our negative core belief: 'I am worthless.'

- **Discussion**
  ○ Relationship between behavioural consequences and protective behaviours
  ○ More examples of their own protective behaviours
  ○ The rules that my protective behaviours support

4 Next week's assignment and end [15 minutes]

Assignment

1 Please complete the table by selecting four activating events. Identify the immediate automatic thoughts and the underlying core beliefs that this event produced. Then describe the protective behaviour you used to cope with your core belief.

Activating Event	Automatic Thought	Core Belief	Protective Behaviour
1			
2			
3			
4			

How we manage our negative core beliefs: rules and protective behaviours

2 Please complete the table by describing the rules that the protective behaviours you listed above support.

Activating Event	Automatic Thought	Core Belief	Protective Behaviour	Rule
1				
2				
3				
4				

3 Please make a list of your post-ABI core beliefs and rules.

My Post-ABI Core Beliefs	My Post-ABI Rules
1	
2	
3	
4	
5	
6	
7	
8	

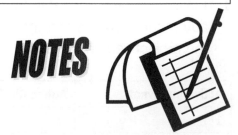

NOTES

What happens when post-ABI rules break down?

Welcome and introduction [10 minutes]

Today's objective

Explore:

1 If all our post-ABI rules are sensible, attainable and realistic
2 If we can uphold all our post-ABI rules at all times
3 What is likely to happen when post-ABI rules break down?

Session outline

1 Summary of last session and assignment review [20 minutes]
2 Group Exercise: Are all post-ABI rules sensible, attainable and realistic; can we uphold them at all times? [40 minutes]
3 Discussion: What happens when post-ABI rules break down? [30 minutes]
4 Next week's assignment and end [15 minutes]

Total time: 115 minutes

1 Summary of last session and assignment review [20 minutes]

2 Are all post-ABI rules sensible, attainable and realistic; can we uphold them at all times? [40 minutes]

What happens when post-ABI rules break down?

 Group Exercise: Please select an activating event from your assignments as a group. Together as a group, please complete either the exercise table or the exercise figure below.

Activating Event	Automatic Thought	Protective Behaviours	Life Rule

Consequence	Emotion	Lifestyle Outcome

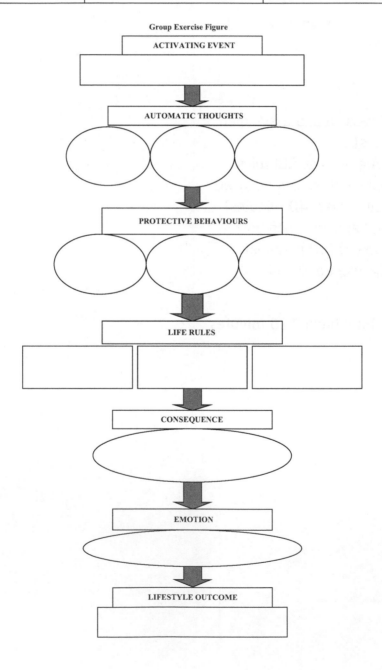

Group Exercise Figure

ACTIVATING EVENT

AUTOMATIC THOUGHTS

PROTECTIVE BEHAVIOURS

LIFE RULES

CONSEQUENCE

EMOTION

LIFESTYLE OUTCOME

What happens when post-ABI rules break down?

- **End Exercise Discussion:**
  - What are the consequences of upholding this rule?
  - What are the lifestyle outcomes of upholding this rule?
  - What are the emotional consequences of upholding this rule?
  - Can I uphold this rule at all times?
  - Does this rule shield me from becoming aware of my negative core beliefs?

- **Exercise Conclusion:** All rules are not sensible, attainable and realistic; we cannot uphold them at all times.

3 Discussion: What happens when post-ABI rules break down? [30 minutes]

- **Reasons for rule break:**
  - Rule standards too high
  - Activating event triggers emotions incompatible with rule
  - Protective behaviours fail to work

- **Vicious circle of rules breakdown:**
  - The **automatic thoughts** overwhelm us
  - **Negative core beliefs** flood in
  - **Negative emotions** follow negative core beliefs
  - Result: **stronger resolve** to reinforce rule with more drastic protective behaviours

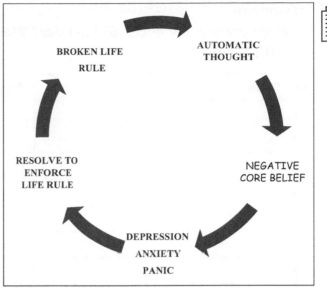

4 Next week's assignment and end [15 minutes]

- What are my key post-ABI life rules? What protective behaviours follow from my life rules?
- What happens when my post-ABI life rules break down?
- Why have my post-ABI rules broken down? (Assignment Table 3)
- What did I do when my post-ABI rules broke down?

What happens when post-ABI rules break down?

Assignment

1 What are my key post-ABI life rules? What protective behaviours follow from my post-ABI life rules?

Life Rules	Protective Behaviours
1	
2	
3	
4	
5	
6	
7	
8	
9	
10	

2 What happens when my post-ABI life rules break down?

Activating Event	Broken Rule	Automatic Thoughts	Negative Core Beliefs	Emotional Consequence

3 Why did my post-ABI rule break down; what did I do when it broke?

Activating Event	Broken Rule	Why Has My Rule Broken Down?	What Did I Do When My Rule Broke Down?

NOTES

Someone to watch over me

Welcome and introduction [10 minutes]

Today's objectives

We will learn:

1   How we process critical events
2   Who watches over us when we face critical events
3   How we can learn to be more effective in managing our emotions and behaviour in the face of critical events

Session outline

1   Summary of last session and assignment review [20 minutes]
2   Processing a critical event: our Watching Self [30 minutes]
3   Exercise: someone to watch over me [15 minutes]
4   Discussion: can we learn to be more effective in managing our emotions and behaviour when faced with critical events? [30 minutes]
5   Next week's assignment and end [15 minutes]

Total time: 120 minutes

1 Summary of last session and assignment review [20 minutes]

2 How do we process a critical event: our Watching Self [30 minutes]

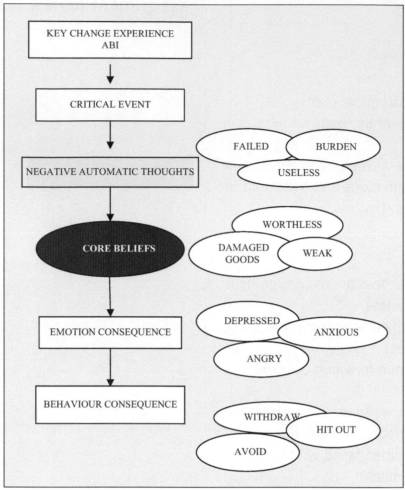

Figure 5.1 Processing critical events

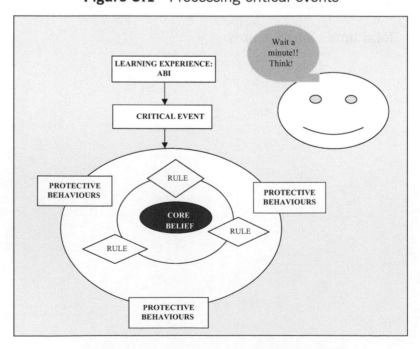

Figure 5.2 Co-opting the watching self

3 Exercise: someone to watch over me [15 minutes]

Please complete the table below by filling the appropriate columns. Think of an activating event, the automatic thoughts it activated and the rules linked to these thoughts. Then try to remember if your Watching Self spoke to you at all to help you manage the situation. If it did not, then write 'NO' in the Watching Self column. State the outcome of the event and the emotions you felt as a result.

Activating Event	Automatic Thoughts	Rule	Did Your Watching Self Speak? What Did It Say?	Outcome	Emotional Consequence
1					
2					
3					
4					
5					
6					

4 Exercise discussion: can we learn to be more effective in managing our emotions and behaviour in the face of critical events? [30 minutes]

5 Next week's assignment and end [15 minutes]

The aim of next week's assignment is to help you learn and remember our discussions of today's session. It is a repeat of this session's exercise and aims to sharpen your awareness of your Watching Self.

ASSIGNMENT

SOMEONE TO WATCH OVER ME: Think of an activating event, the automatic thoughts it activated and the rules linked to these thoughts. Then try to remember if your Watching Self intervened to help you manage the situation. State the outcome of the event and the emotions you felt as a result. Complete the table below by filling the appropriate columns.

Activating Event	Automatic Thoughts	Rule	Did Your Watching Self Speak? What Did It Say?	Outcome	Emotional Consequence

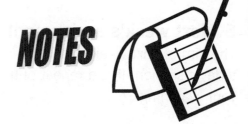

NOTES

MODULE 3

Mastering change

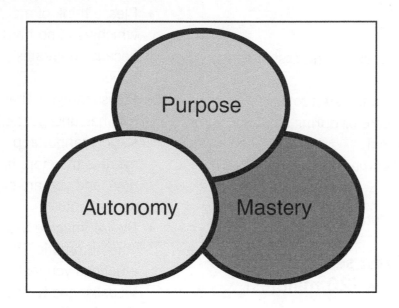

Breaking rules voluntarily

Welcome and introduction [5 minutes]

Today's objective

We will learn to:

Become aware of our Watching Self when faced with critical events

Session outline

1 Summary of last session and assignment review [20 minutes]
2 Become aware of and listen to our Watching Self before or during a critical event: [70 minutes]
3 Next week's assignment and end [15 minutes]

Total time: 110 minutes

1 Summary of last session and assignment review [20 minutes]

2 Become aware of and listen to our Watching Self before and during a critical event [70 minutes]

- 'On-line processing' engulfs us and leads us to make rigid interpretations about ourselves, others and the world. We believe these to be 'true'
- 'On-line processing' makes us feel as though we might lose control

○ **EXERCISE 1: Breaking rules 'cold' during a critical event: CONSEQUENCES [15 minutes]**

- ♦ Please think of a critical event which you find hard to cope with because it creates painful emotions in you.
- ♦ Please imagine that your protective rule has unexpectedly broken down so you cannot apply it. This critical event is therefore happening here and now, and you are experiencing it this very minute.
- ♦ Please imagine the critical event, your automatic thoughts and the emotions you feel very vividly. Visualise the full scenario in detail. Complete the table below, also stating the unexpectedly broken rule which you cannot apply. I have given an example.
- ♦ You have 1 minute's imagination time and 15 minutes to record the vivid scenes you have imagined.

Breaking rules voluntarily

Table 1 EXERCISE 1

Rule	Activating Event	Automatic Thought	Rule Break Emotional Consequence
EXAMPLE: Always give self a lot more time than I need so I can make sure I get there on time and have time to settle down	Left 40 minutes earlier than needed but bus drivers were on strike, and I had to walk to another bus stop 20 minutes away to catch a bus; I had to wait for 10 minutes for a bus to come	Will be late for appointment Will be late for dinner Will be told off Will miss bus back Bus will not arrive Traffic will be bad I will be made a fool of Just my luck	Panic; disaster

○ **DISCUSSION [20 minutes]**

○ **EXERCISE 2: breaking rules voluntarily with the support of Watching Self before or during a critical event: consequences [15 minutes]**

♦ Now please think of the same critical event but imagine yourself thinking it through and discussing it with your Watching Self as it happens. Please ensure your visualisation of the scenario and of your conversation with your Watching Self is very vivid, as if the whole scene were happening here and now.

♦ Complete the table below. I have given an example. [1 minute imagination time; 15 minutes recording time]

Table 2 EXERCISE 2

Rule	Rule Break Activating Event	Automatic Thought	Expected Outcome	What Does Your Watching Self Say?	Desired Outcome
EXAMPLE: Always give self a lot more time than I need so I can make sure I get there on time and have time to settle down	Left 40 minutes earlier than needed but bus drivers were on strike and I had to walk to another bus stop 20 minutes away to catch a bus; I had to wait for 10 minutes for a bus to come	Will be late for appointment Will be late for dinner Will be told off Will miss bus back Bus will not arrive Traffic will be bad I will be made a fool of Just my luck	Panic; disaster	Appointment venue only 15 minutes away; unlikely to be late If late explain the situation: reason is perfectly legitimate How likely is it that they will tell me off? As an adult no one can tell me off If people tell me off, I tell them calmly they are being illogical If bus does not come, I can reschedule appointment	I will not be late If I am late, I can deal with it People are very unlikely to tell me off If people told me off, I would tell them I expect them to be civil If people are rude to me, I can take my custom elsewhere

Breaking rules voluntarily

Rule	Rule Break Activating Event	Automatic Thought	Expected Outcome	What Does Your Watching Self Say?	Desired Outcome

○ **DISCUSSION [20 minutes]**

3 Next week's assignment and end [15 minutes]

Please do Exercise 2 again but use a different scenario. Remember to use your imagination to visualise the scenario and your conversation with your Watching Self very vividly, as if you were experiencing the whole scene here and now.

Complete the table below

Rule	Rule Break Activating Event	Automatic Thought	Expected Outcome	What Does Your Watching Self Say?	Desired Outcome

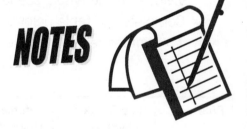

NOTES

Breaking rules voluntarily: confronting our fears, learning to be boss

Welcome and introduction [5 minutes]

Today's objective:

Gaining control of our fears by confronting them and by learning to:

1 Enter a state of relaxation
2 Imagine vividly our fear-provoking critical events whilst in a state of relaxation
3 Imagine that we are experiencing our fear-provoking critical events here and now
4 Allow ourselves to feel negative emotions whilst imagining that we are experiencing our fear-provoking critical events here and now
5 Listen to our Watching Self to manage negative emotions and to generate solutions to the problems that our critical events present

Session outline

1 Summary of last session and assignment review [20 minutes]
2 Learning to enter a state of relaxation [15 minutes]
3 Imagining that we are experiencing our fear-provoking critical events here and now and allowing ourselves to feel negative emotions [50 minutes]
4 Feedback [15 minutes]
5 Next week's assignment and end [10 minutes]

Total time: 110 minutes

1 Summary of last session and assignment review [20 minutes]

2 Learning to enter a state of relaxation [15 minutes]

The key five learning points of relaxation training:

1 Reinforcement mechanism that maintains our dysfunctional rules

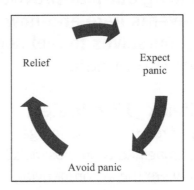

2 Characteristics of SMART scenarios and selection of critical events for exposure

Not Smart	Smart
Fear of failure Fear of causing disappointment Fear of causing displeasure	Making a specific mistake on a specific assignment Letting someone down on a specific promise you have made or a specific expectation they have about you; Refusing to carry out a specific request
Fear of losing control Fear of being a burden Fear of being/being perceived as inadequate	A specific instance of involuntary rule break; dropping plate of food on kitchen floor Causing a specific row or disagreement; making a specific error Being challenged in a specific situation by a specific issue
Fear of danger	Being in a specific situation perceived as risky; football match, concert

3 Communicating whilst in a relaxed state: signalling

Breaking rules voluntarily: confronting our fears, learning to be boss

4 Making relaxation work
5 Developing the skills to self-relax

3 Imagining that we are experiencing our fear-provoking critical events here and now and allowing ourselves to feel negative emotions [50 minutes]

4 Feedback [15 minutes]

- Quality of relaxation and imagery:
  - Were imagined scenarios vivid?
  - What were the accompanying emotions?

- Watching Self:
  - Did Watching Self help manage negative emotions effectively?
  - Did Watching Self offer constructive solutions to the problems posed by critical events?

- Safe place
  - Was retreat to safe place relaxing? Helpful?

5 Next week's assignment and end [10 minutes]

Three assignments:

1 **Rehearsal:** Practise this session's recorded relaxation exercise in full as recorded at least three times during the week
2 **Behavioural experiment:** Trial the imagined critical event in real-life at least three times during the week
3 **Recording:** Record the outcome in the two assignment tables [next pages] handout

Please remember to bring recording devices, pillows and scarves for next week's relaxation exercise

Breaking rules voluntarily: confronting our fears, learning to be boss

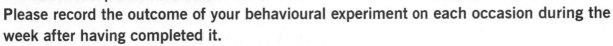

Behavioural experiment tables
Please record the outcome of your behavioural experiment on each occasion during the week after having completed it.

Date:

Critical Event Scenario	Violated Rule	Automatic Thoughts	What Did I Feel During Behavioural Experiment?	How Did My Watching Self Help Me Manage the Situation?	Outcome	What Did I Feel at End of Behavioural Experiment?

Date:

Critical Event Scenario	Violated Rule	Automatic Thoughts	What Did I Feel During Behavioural Experiment?	How Did My Watching Self Help Me Manage the Situation?	Outcome	What Did I Feel at End of Behavioural Experiment?

Date:

Critical Event Scenario	Violated Rule	Automatic Thoughts	What Did I Feel During Behavioural Experiment?	How Did My Watching Self Help Me Manage the Situation?	Outcome	What Did I Feel at End of Behavioural Experiment?

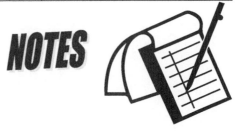

Are our negative beliefs about ourselves true?

Welcome and introduction [5 minutes]

Today's objectives:

1 Extend our mastery over critical events
2 Learn that effective coping is mastery of critical events
3 Prepare to evaluate our core beliefs

Session outline

1 Summary of last session and assignment review [20 minutes]
2 Relaxation/imaginary exposure to a new set of critical events [50 minutes]
3 Group feedback [20 minutes]
4 Group discussion: are our negative beliefs about ourselves true; should we keep our life rules? [25 minutes]
5 Next week's assignment and end [10 minutes]

Total time: 125 minutes

1 Summary of last session and assignment review [20 minutes]

2 Relaxation/imaginary exposure to a new set of critical events [50 minutes]

3 Group feedback [20 minutes]

Comparison of this session's imaginary exposure with that of the last session and that of home-rehearsal in terms of:

- Quality of relaxation and imagery:
  ○ Were imagined scenarios vivid?
  ○ What were the accompanying emotions?

- Watching Self:
  ○ Did Watching Self help manage negative emotions effectively?
  ○ Did Watching Self offer constructive solutions to the problems posed by critical events?

- Safe place
  ○ Was retreat to safe place relaxing? Helpful?

Are our negative beliefs about ourselves true?

4 Group discussion: are our negative beliefs about ourselves true? [25 minutes]

- Recalling my negative core beliefs
- Selecting two negative core beliefs
- Rating the evidence for it and the evidence against it

Negative Core Belief 1		Negative Core Belief 2	
Evidence For	Evidence Against	Evidence For	Evidence Against
1	1	1	1
2	2	2	2
3	3	3	3
4	4	4	4
5	5	5	5
6	6	6	6

5 Next week's assignment and end [10 minutes]

Four assignments:

1 **Rehearsal:** Practise this session's recorded relaxation exercise in full as recorded at least three times during the week
2 **Behavioural experiment:** Trial the imagined critical event in real-life at least three times during the week
3 **Recording:** Record the outcome in the assignment table in the handout
4 **Evaluating negative core beliefs:** Select two negative core beliefs and rate the evidence for them and against them in light of your achievements in the last four sessions

Assignment sheets
Behavioural experiment recording tables

Critical Event Scenario	Violated Rule	Automatic Thoughts	What Did I Feel During Behavioural Experiment?	How Did My Watching Self Help Me Manage the Situation?	Outcome	What Did I Feel at End of Behavioural Experiment?

Are our negative beliefs about ourselves true?

 Please record the outcome of your behavioural experiment on each occasion during the week after having completed it.

Date:

Critical Event Scenario	Violated Rule	Automatic Thoughts	What Did I Feel During Behavioural Experiment?	How Did My Watching Self Help Me Manage the Situation?	Outcome	What Did I Feel at End of Behavioural Experiment?

Date:

Critical Event Scenario	Violated Rule	Automatic Thoughts	What Did I Feel During Behavioural Experiment?	How Did My Watching Self Help Me Manage the Situation?	Outcome	What Did I Feel at End of Behavioural Experiment?

EVALUATING MY NEGATIVE CORE BELIEFS

Please select two negative core beliefs and rate the evidence for and against them

Negative Core Belief 1		Negative Core Belief 2	
Evidence For It	Evidence Against It	Evidence For It	Evidence Against It
1	1	1	1
2	2	2	2
3	3	3	3
4	4	4	4
5	5	5	5
6	6	6	6
7	7	7	7
8	8	8	8

NOTES

Evidence for our beliefs and our rules

Welcome and introduction [5 minutes]

Today's objective:

To realise that:

1 We can exercise control over situations we perceive as threatening by mastering a wider range of critical events
2 We are able to attain our goals by making our recent achievements a central part of our post-ABI belief and rule systems

Session outline

1 Summary of last session and assignment review [20 minutes]
2 Group discussion of the results of our assignment in the context of the goals we have attained [35 minutes]
3 Group exercise: rating the consequences of one of our post-ABI dysfunctional life rules [35 minutes]
4 Next week's assignment and end [10 minutes]

Total time: 105 minutes

1 Summary of last session and assignment review [20 minutes]

2 Group discussion of the results of our assignment in the context of the goals we have attained [35 minutes]

Evidence for our beliefs and our rules

Table 1 Behavioural experiment goal and achievement

Shared Goal	Shared Achievement Yes/No	Was I Able To Engage in These Activites Before the Group Programme?
Be comfortable in crowded places [example]		

Table 2 Shared negative core belief evaluation

Shared Belief	Belief Is Not True of Me Now [X]	Belief Is Still True of Me [X]
I am faulty goods [example]		

3 Group exercise: rating the consequences of one of our post-ABI dysfunctional life rules [35 minutes]

Table 3 Analysing the consequences of a shared life rule

Life Rule	Negative Consequences of Adhering to Rule	Positive Consequences of Rule Break	Should We Maintain This Rule?

4 Next week's assignment and end [10 minutes]

This is the programme's last assignment in preparation for next week's last session.

Evidence for our beliefs and our rules

Four assignments:

1 **Rehearsal:** Practise the recorded relaxation exercise in full with a new set of critical event scenarios
2 **Behavioural experiment:** Trial the imagined new critical event in real-life at least three times during the week
3 **Recording:** Record the Behavioural Experiment outcome in the assignment table in the handout
4 **Evaluating dysfunctional life rules:** Select two dysfunctional life rules and identify the negative consequences of adhering to them and the positive consequences of breaking them

Assignment sheets
Behavioural experiment recording tables

Critical Event Scenario	Violated Rule	Automatic Thoughts	What Did I Feel During Behavioural Experiment?	How Did My Watching Self Help Me Manage the Situation?	Outcome	What Did I Feel at End of Behavioural Experiment?

Please record the outcome of your behavioural experiment on each occasion during the week after having completed it.

Date:

Critical Event Scenario	Violated Rule	Automatic Thoughts	What Did I Feel During Behavioural Experiment?	How Did My Watching Self Help Me Manage the Situation?	Outcome	What Did I Feel at End of Behavioural Experiment?

Evidence for our beliefs and our rules

Date:

Critical Event Scenario	Violated Rule	Automatic Thoughts	What Did I Feel During Behavioural Experiment?	How Did My Watching Self Help Me Manage the Situation?	Outcome	What Did I Feel at End of Behavioural Experiment?

Evaluating the consequences of two of my dysfunctional life rules:

Please select two dysfunctional life rules and identify the negative consequences of adhering to them and the positive consequences of breaking them.

Life Rules	Negative Consequences of Adhering to Rule	Positive Consequences of Rule Break	Should We Maintain This Rule?
1 2			

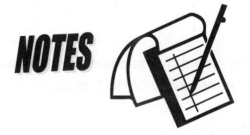

Goodbye: ABI – a life-long learning experience

Welcome and introduction [5 minutes]

Today's objective:

To consolidate and enduringly retain the learning gains we have achieved throughout the programme.

Session outline

1 Summary of last session and assignment review [20 minutes]
2 Life-long practice of relaxation/imaginary exposure and behaviour experiments whenever critical events face us [10 minutes]
3 Group discussion: key learning points of the programme's three modules [30 minutes]
4 Group discussion: recognising our own self-efficacy [35 minutes]
5 Goodbye: ABI – a life-long learning experience [20 minutes]

Total time: 115 minutes

1 Summary of last session and assignment review [20 minutes]

2 Life-long practice of relaxation/ imaginary exposure and behaviour experiments whenever critical events face us [10 minutes]

3 Group discussion: the key learning points of the programme's three modules [30 minutes]

Goodbye: ABI – a life-long learning experience

Table 1   Key learning points of programme modules

Modules	What Did We Do?	What Did We Learn?	Key Learning Points
1 Recognising change			
2 Exploring change			
3 Mastering change			

4 Group discussion: recognising our own self-efficacy [35 minutes]

Table 2   Examples of self-efficacy from Module 3 key learning points

Key Learning Points From Module 3	Examples of Recent Self-Efficacy	Examples of Lifetime Self-Efficacy
•		
•		
•		

5 ABI: a life-long learning experience [20 minutes]

How do we define our ABI experience?

ABI is such a momentous, frame-breaking experience that it remains a life-long active learning benchmark against which to measure almost all of life's other critical incidents.

GOODBYE

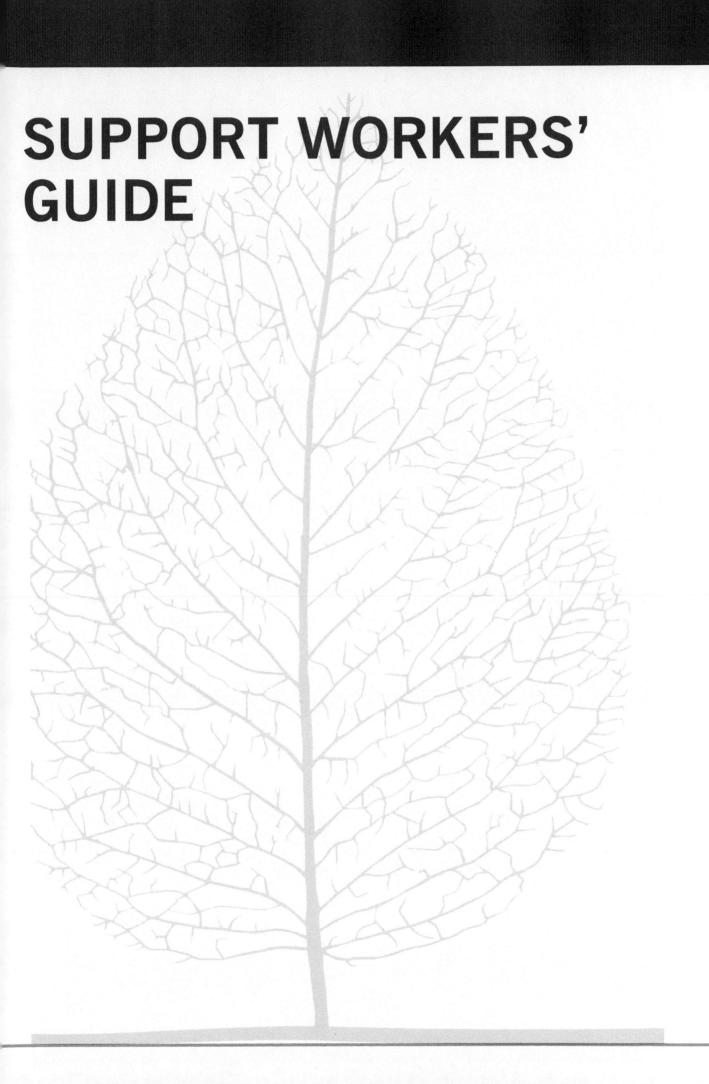

SUPPORT WORKERS' GUIDE

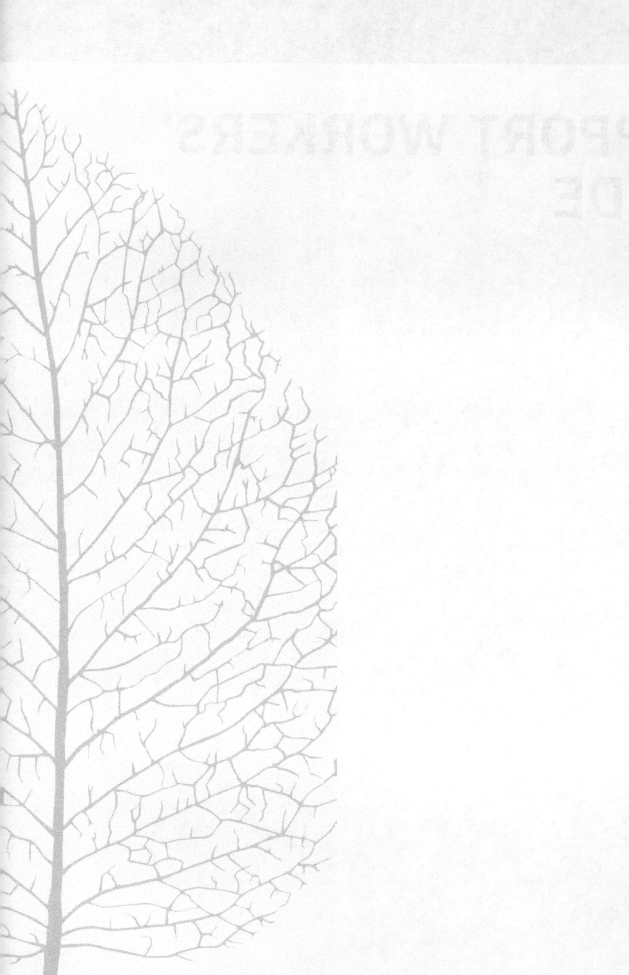

MODULE 1

Recognising change

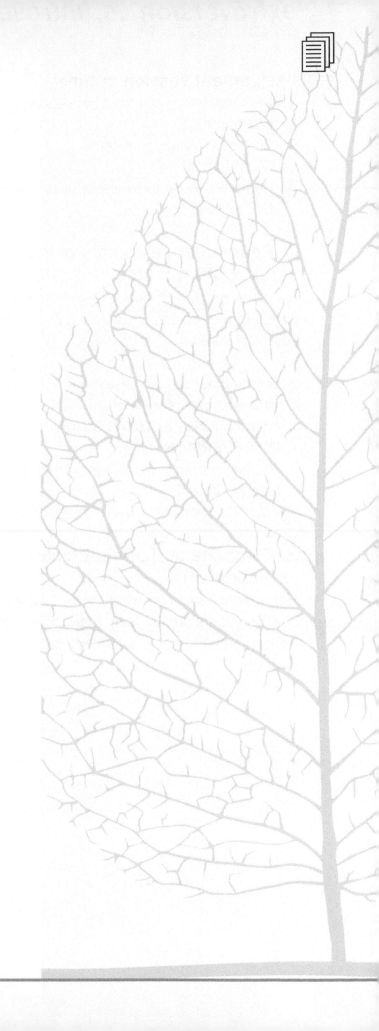

How do I make relationships? extroversion vs. introversion

Assignment session outline[1]

1 Remember key points of the session [20 minutes]
2 Complete assignment tables [20 minutes]
3 Complete feedback questionnaire [20 minutes]

1 Remember key points of the session [20 minutes]

Help/prompt participants to recall the key points of the session in their own words. The key points were:

- Learning about how they made relationships before their ABI and after their ABI: **EXTROVERSION** vs. **INTROVERSION**
- The key changes they have experienced before and after
- What did they think were the reasons?

2 Complete assignment tables [20 minutes]

Help participants complete Tables 1, 2 and 3. Participants should keep their completed assignments in their session logs filed under the appropriate session. Answer any questions but do not influence ratings.

During assignment completion time, draw three tables on the flip chart as shown on the next page. After participants complete their assignment, ask them to read out their ratings and note them on the flip chart. Discuss their results with the group.

Copy flip-chart content in your notes.

3 Complete feedback questionnaire [20 minutes]

Ask participants to complete the feedback questionnaire. Answer any questions but do not influence ratings. Remember, participants are likely to disagree with a number of questions relating to activities of daily and community living, and there may not be any examples given for these activities. Reassure them by telling them that it is perfectly acceptable to disagree with some of the statements of the questionnaire. Collect the questionnaires upon completion.

How do I make relationships? extroversion vs. introversion

Assignment Table 1

Participant[2]	After ABI		Before ABI	
	Extrovert	Introvert	Extrovert	Introvert
1				
2				
3				
4				
5				
6				
7				
8				
TOTAL				

Assignment Table 2   How has the way I make relationships changed?

	Me After My ABI	Me Before My ABI
1		
2		
3		
4		
5		

Assignment Table 3

What Do I Want to Change About the Way I Make Relationships After My ABI?
1
2
3
4
5
6
7

How do I gather information? sensing vs. intuition

Assignment session outline
1 Remember key points of the session
2 Complete assignment tables
3 Complete feedback questionnaire

1 Remember key points of the session [20 minutes]

Help/prompt participants to recall the key points of the session in their own words. The key points were:

- Learning about the importance of information gathering
- Learning about how they gathered information before their ABI and after their ABI: **SENSING** vs. **INTUITION**
- The key changes they have experienced before and after
- What did they think were the reasons?

2 Complete assignment tables [20 minutes]

Help participants complete Tables 1, 2 and 3. Participants should keep their completed assignments in their session logs filed under the appropriate session. Answer any questions but do not influence ratings.

During assignment completion time, draw three tables on the flip chart as shown on the next page. After participants have completed their assignment, ask them to read out their ratings and note them on the flip chart. Facilitate group discussion of results.

Copy flip-chart content in your notes.

3 Complete feedback questionnaire [20 minutes]

Ask participants to complete the feedback questionnaire. Answer any questions but do not influence ratings. Remember, participants are likely to disagree with a number of questions relating to activities of daily and community living, and there are not going to be any examples given for these activities. Reassure them by telling them that it is perfectly acceptable to disagree with some of the statements of the questionnaire. Collect the questionnaires upon completion.

How do I gather information?
sensing vs. intuition

Assignment Table 1

Participant	After ABI		Before ABI	
	Sensing	Intuition	Sensing	Intuition
1				
2				
3				
4				
5				
6				
7				
TOTAL				

Assignment Table 2   How has my information gathering changed?

	Me After My ABI	Me Before My ABI
1		
2		
3		
4		
5		
6		
7		

Assignment Table 3

What Do I Want to Change About My Information Gathering After My ABI?
1
2
3
4
5
6
7
8

How do I make decisions? thinking vs. feeling

Assignment session outline

1 Remember key points of the session
2 Complete assignment tables
3 Complete feedback questionnaire

1 Remember key points of the session [20 minutes]

Help/prompt participants to recall the key points of the session in their own words. The key points were:

- Learning about how they made decisions before their ABI and after their ABI: **THINKING** vs. **FEELING**
- The key changes they have experienced before and after
- What did they think were the reasons?

2 Complete assignment tables [20 minutes]

Help participants complete Tables 1, 2 and 3. Participants should keep their completed assignments in their session logs filed under the appropriate session. Answer any questions but do not influence ratings.

During assignment completion time, draw three tables on the flip chart as shown on the next page. After participants have completed their assignment, ask them to read out their ratings and note them on the flip chart. Facilitate group discussion of results.

Copy flip-chart content in your notes.

3 Complete feedback questionnaire [20 minutes]

Ask participants to complete the feedback questionnaire. Answer any questions but do not influence ratings. Remember, participants are likely to disagree with a number of questions relating to activities of daily and community living, and there may not be any examples given for these activities. Reassure them by telling them that it is perfectly acceptable to disagree with some of the statements of the questionnaire. Collect the questionnaires upon completion.

How do I make decisions?
thinking vs. feeling

Assignment Table 1

Participant	After ABI		Before ABI	
	Thinking	Feeling	Thinking	Feeling
1				
2				
3				
4				
5				
6				
7				
TOTAL				

Assignment Table 2   How has my decision-making changed?

	Me After My ABI	Me Before My ABI
1		
2		
3		
4		
5		
6		
7		

Assignment Table 3

What Do I Want To Change About My Decision-Making After My ABI?
1
2
3
4
5
6
7
8

How do I organise my life?
judging vs. perceiving

Assignment session outline
1 **Remember key points of the session**
2 **Complete assignment tables**
3 **Complete feedback questionnaire**

1 Remember key points of the session [20 minutes]
Help/prompt participants to recall the key points of the session in their own words. The key points were:

- Learning about lifestyle: what people see about them and their lives.
- Learning about the changes that occurred in their lifestyles post-ABI.
- What did they think were the reasons?

2 Complete assignment tables [30 minutes]
Help participants to complete assignment Tables 1 and 2. Participants should keep their completed assignments in their session logs filed under the appropriate session. Answer any questions but do not influence ratings.

When you get to the third assignment, help participants go through their session logs and pick out their pre- and post-ABI preferences on all four dimensions. Help them to note these dimensions on Assignment Table 3. Facilitate a 10-minute discussion on the reasons for any pre- and post-ABI differences. Explore the changes they wish to make in their post-ABI preferences.

Help participants complete Assignment Tables 4 and 5.

During assignment completion time, draw four tables on the flip chart, combining Assignment Tables 3 and 4, as shown on pages 2 and 3. After participants have completed their assignments, ask them to read out their ratings and note them on the flip chart. Facilitate group discussion of results.

Copy flip-chart content in your notes.

How do I organise my life?
judging vs. perceiving

Assignment Table 1

Participant	After ABI		Before ABI	
	Judging	Perceiving	Judging	Perceiving
1				
2				
3				
4				
5				
6				
7				
TOTAL				

Assignment Table 2   How my lifestyle has changed

	Me After My ABI	Me Before My ABI
1		
2		
3		
4		
5		
6		
7		

Assignment Tables 3 and 4   [combined]

	Preference Pre-ABI								Preference Post-ABI								Pre-ABI	Post-ABI
	E	I	S	N	T	F	J	P	E	I	S	N	T	F	J	P	Type	Type
1																		
2																		
3																		
4																		
5																		
6																		
7																		
TOTAL																		

How do I organise my life?
judging vs. perceiving

Assignment Table 5

	Pre-ABI	Post-ABI	Short Description of How I Have Changed	Which of My Post-Abi Preferences Do I Wish to Change?
	Type	Type		
1				
2				
3				
4				
5				
6				
7				

3 Complete evaluation questionnaire [20 minutes]

Ask participants to complete the feedback questionnaire. Answer any questions but do not influence ratings. Remember, participants are likely to disagree with a number of questions relating to activities of daily and community living, and there may not be any examples given for these activities. Reassure them by telling them that it is perfectly acceptable to disagree with some of the statements of the questionnaire. Collect the questionnaires upon completion.

Notes

1 Take notes of all proceedings during the session including the contents of the flip chart. At the end of the session, collect all materials and documents and hand them to the group practitioner well before the next group session.
2 Names have been replaced by numbers.

MODULE 2

Exploring change

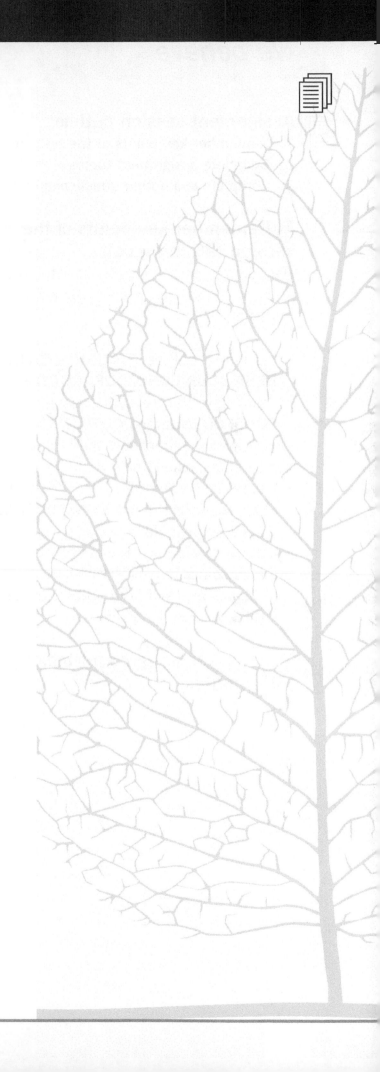

How we think impacts how we behave

Assignment session outline[1]
1 Remember key points of the session
2 Complete assignment tables
3 Complete evaluation questionnaire

1 Remember key points of the session [20 minutes]
Help/prompt participants to recall the key points of the session in their own words. The key points were:

- Learning about the **THOUGHT-FEELING-BEHAVIOUR CONSEQUENCE CYLE**
- Learning the difference between **CONSEQUENCE** and **OUTCOME**
- Identifying the impact of their thoughts on their emotions and behaviour
- Identifying the impact of their **THOUGHT-FEELING-BEHAVIOUR CONSEQUENCE CYLES** on their life quality
- Proposing solutions on ways of improving the outcomes of their THOUGHT-FEELING-BEHAVIOUR CONSEQUENCE CYLES on their life quality

2 Complete assignment tables [30 minutes]
This session's assignments are slightly more complex. Participants are likely to need more help from you. It may be more difficult for them to find five thought examples to complete assignment Table 1. They may find it difficult to identify and put into words how they feel about the outcomes in assignment Table 2. Identifying solutions to improve outcomes may also be challenging for them. Help participants accomplish these tasks by facilitating discussion, stimulating their recall and guiding their thinking.

Participants should keep their completed assignments in their session logs filed under the appropriate session. Answer any questions but do not influence ratings.

During assignment completion time, draw three tables on the flip chart, as shown on pages 2–5.[2] After participants have completed their assignment, ask them to read out their statements and note them on the flip chart. Facilitate group discussion of results.

Assignment Table 1

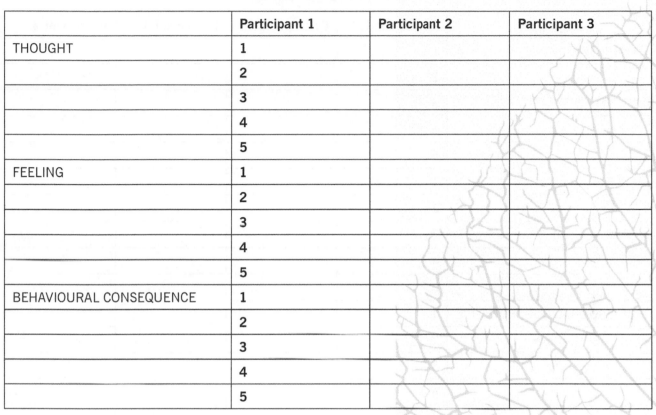

		Participant 1	Participant 2	Participant 3
THOUGHT	1			
	2			
	3			
	4			
	5			
FEELING	1			
	2			
	3			
	4			
	5			
BEHAVIOURAL CONSEQUENCE	1			
	2			
	3			
	4			
	5			

		Participant 4	Participant 5	Participant 6	Participant 7
THOUGHT	1				
	2				
	3				
	4				
	5				
FEELING	1				
	2				
	3				
	4				
	5				
BEHAVIOURAL CONSEQUENCE	1				
	2				
	3				
	4				
	5				

Assignment Table 2

		Participant 1	Participant 2	Participant 3	Participant 4
THOUGHT	1				
	2				
	3				
	4				
	5				
FEELING	1				
	2				
	3				
	4				
	5				
BEHAVIOURAL CONSEQUENCE	1				
	2				
	3				
	4				
	5				
OUTCOME	1				
	2				
	3				
	4				
	5				
EMOTION ABOUT OUTCOME	1				
	2				
	3				
	4				
	5				

		Participant 5	Participant 6	Participant 7
THOUGHT	1			
	2			
	3			
	4			

(Continued)

Assignment Table 2 (Continued)

	5		
FEELING	1		
	2		
	3		
	4		
	5		
BEHAVIOURAL CONSEQUENCE	1		
	2		
	3		
	4		
	5		
OUTCOME	1		
	2		
	3		
	4		
	5		
EMOTION ABOUT OUTCOME	1		
	2		
	3		
	4		
	5		

Assignment Table 3

		Participant 1	Participant 2	Participant 3	Participant 4
OUTCOME	1				
	2				
	3				
	4				
	5				

(Continued)

Assignment Table 3 (Continued)

		Participant 1	Participant 2	Participant 3	Participant 4
HOW CAN I CHANGE THIS OUTCOME?	1				
	2				
	3				
	4				
	5				
		Participant 5	Participant 6	Participant 7	Participant 8
OUTCOME	1				
	2				
	3				
	4				
	5				
HOW CAN I CHANGE THIS OUTCOME?	1				
	2				
	3				
	4				
	5				

3 Complete evaluation questionnaire [20 minutes]

Ask participants to complete the feedback questionnaire. Answer any questions but do not influence ratings. Remember, participants are likely to disagree with a number of questions relating to activities of daily and community living, and there may not be any examples given for these activities. Reassure them by telling them that it is perfectly acceptable to disagree with some of the statements of the questionnaire. Collect the questionnaires upon completion.

How we think impacts how we behave: automatic thoughts before/after ABI

Assignment session outline
1 Remember key points of the session
2 Complete assignment tables
3 Complete evaluation questionnaire

1 Remember key points of the session [20 minutes]
Help/prompt participants to recall the key points of the session in their own words. The key points were:

- Description of automatic thoughts
- Identifying differences in pre- and post-ABI automatic thoughts
- Introducing the concept of core beliefs as the basis of automatic thoughts

2 Complete assignment tables [30 minutes]
Participants may need your help in completing the first two assignment tables. Their key difficulties are likely to be in

1 Rating the negative quality of their post- and pre-ABI feelings generated by their automatic thoughts in Assignment Table 1
2 Identifying the core beliefs underlying their post-ABI automatic thoughts in Assignment Table 2

Making a list of their core beliefs in Table 3 should not be too onerous a task, but participants may need your help with this also.

Participants should keep their completed assignments in their session logs filed under the appropriate session. Answer any questions but do not influence ratings.

During assignment completion time, draw three tables on the flip chart, as shown on pages 2–3. After participants have completed their assignment, ask them to read out their statements and note them on the flip chart. Facilitate group discussion of results.

Copy flip-chart content in your notes.

How we think impacts how we behave: automatic thoughts before/after ABI

Assignment Table 1A   Pre-ABI

		Participant 1	Participant 2	Participant 3	Participant 4
ACTIVATING EVENT	1				
	2				
	3				
AUTOMATIC THOUGHT	1				
	2				
	3				
FEELING RATING	1				
	2				
	3				

Assignment Table 1B   Post-ABI

		Participant 1	Participant 2	Participant 3	Participant 4
ACTIVATING EVENT	1				
	2				
	3				
AUTOMATIC THOUGHT	1				
	2				
	3				
FEELING RATING	1				
	2				
	3				

Assignment Table 2   Core beliefs

		Participant 1	Participant 2	Participant 3	Participant 4
ACTIVATING EVENT	1				
	2				
	3				

How we think impacts how we behave: automatic thoughts before/after ABI

AUTOMATIC THOUGHT	1			
	2			
	3			
CORE BELIEF	1			
	2			
	3			

Assignment Table 3 Core belief list

	Participant 1	Participant 2	Participant 3	Participant 4
CORE BELIEFS				

3 Complete evaluation questionnaire [20 minutes]

Ask participants to complete the feedback questionnaire. Answer any questions but do not influence ratings. Remember, participants are likely to disagree with a number of questions relating to activities of daily and community living, and there may not be any examples given for these activities. Reassure them by telling them that it is perfectly acceptable to disagree with some of the statements of the questionnaire. Collect the questionnaires upon completion.

How we manage our negative core beliefs: rules and protective behaviours

Assignment session outline
1 Remember key points of the session
2 Complete assignment tables
3 Complete evaluation questionnaire

1 Remember key points of the session [20 minutes]

Help/prompt participants to recall the key points of the session in their own words. The key points were:

- Behavioural consequences are coping mechanisms
- Coping mechanisms are protective behaviours that shield us from painful core beliefs
- Protective behaviours support a series of rules we have devised to shield us from our painful core beliefs

2 Complete assignment tables [30 minutes]

Participants may need your help in completing the assignment tables despite the practice they have received during the session. In particular, they may find it difficult to extrapolate rules from protective behaviours. For example, the protective behaviour and rule associated with the post-ABI preference change from introversion to extroversion may be as shown in the example on the table on next page:

How we manage our negative core beliefs: rules and protective behaviours

Assignment Table 1

Activating Event	Core Belief	Behavioural Consequence/ Protective Behaviour	Rule
Invited to a party with many people I don't know	They will think me stupid [because I can't find the right words]	Refuse invitation	If I avoid meeting people I don't know, they will not think me stupid

Refer to the session discussions and exercise to help them with the assignment.

Participants should keep their completed assignments in their session logs filed under the appropriate session. Answer any questions but do not influence ratings.

During assignment completion time, draw two tables on flip chart, as shown below. After participants have completed their assignment, ask them to read out their statements and note them on the flip chart. Facilitate group discussion of results.

Assignment Table 2 Core beliefs

		Participant 1	Participant 2	Participant 3	Participant 4
ACTIVATING EVENT	1				
	2				
	3				
CORE BELIEF	1				
	2				
	3				
PROTECTIVE BEHAVIOUR	1				
	2				
	3				
RULE	1				
	2				
	3				

Assignment Table 3 Rule list

	Participant 1	Participant 2	Participant 3	Participant 4
RULES				

3 Complete evaluation questionnaire [20 minutes]

Ask participants to complete the feedback questionnaire. Answer any questions but do not
influence ratings. Remember, participants are likely to disagree with a number of questions
relating to activities of daily and community living, and there may not be any examples given
for these activities. Reassure them by telling them that it is perfectly acceptable to disagree
with some of the statements of the questionnaire. Collect the questionnaires upon completion.

What happens when post-ABI rules break down?

Assignment session outline
1 Remember key points of the session
2 Complete assignment tables
3 Complete evaluation questionnaire

1 Remember key points of the session [20 minutes]

Help/prompt participants to recall the key points of the session in their own words. The key points were:

- Many of our post-ABI rules and protective behaviours are not sensible and realistic because we cannot uphold them at all times
- Rules break down in uncontrolled, unexpected situations
- Most of our post-ABI rules and protective behaviours are therefore dysfunctional because they do not achieve the purposes we want them to achieve

2 Complete assignment tables [30 minutes]

Participants may need your help in completing the assignment tables despite

the practice they have received during the session. In particular, they may find it difficult to extrapolate protective behaviours from rules, to recall what happened when a rule broke down and what they did in that event.

Refer to the session discussions and exercise to help them with the assignment.

Participants should keep their completed assignments in their session logs filed under the appropriate session. Answer any questions but do not influence ratings.

During assignment completion time, draw three tables on the flip chart, as shown below. After participants have completed their assignment, ask them to read out their statements and note them on the flip chart. Facilitate group discussion of results.

What happens when post-ABI rules break down?

Assignment Table 1

Participant 1		Participant 2		Participant 3		Participant 4		Participant 5	
Rules	Protect Behav	Rules	Protect Behav	Rules	Protect Behav	Rules	Protect Behav	Rules	Protect Behav

Assignment Table 2 Core beliefs

		Participant 1	Participant 2	Participant 3	Participant 4
ACTIVATING EVENT	1				
	2				
	3				
BROKEN RULE	1				
	2				
	3				
AUTOMATIC THOUGHT	1				
	2				
	3				
NEGATIVE CORE BELIEF	1				
	2				
	3				
EMOTIONAL CONSEQUENCE	1				
	2				
	3				

Assignment Table 3

	Broken Rule	Why Did It Break?	What Did I Do When Rule Broke?
1			
2			
3			
4			
5			

3 Complete evaluation questionnaire [20 minutes]

Ask participants to complete the feedback questionnaire. Answer any questions but do not influence ratings. Remember, participants may disagree with a number of questions relating to activities of daily and community living, and there may not be any examples given for these activities. Reassure them by telling them that it is perfectly acceptable to disagree with some of the statements of the questionnaire. Collect the questionnaires upon completion.

Someone to watch over me

Assignment session outline

1 Remember key points of the session
2 Complete assignment table
3 Complete evaluation questionnaire

1 Remember key points of the session [20 minutes]

Help/prompt participants to recall the key points of the session in their own words. The key points were:

- On-line processing is when you are immersed in the emotion of the activating event
- Your Watching Self helps you to manage the situation by creating a distance between you and the critical event so you can think straight. It helps you to assess yourself in relation to it
- A good analogy is a tummy upset
- Your exercise results show that some of you are aware of your Watching Self
- Next week's assignment aims to sharpen your awareness of your Watching Self

2 Complete assignment tables [30 minutes]

Participants may need your help in completing the assignment tables despite the practice they have received during the session. Refer to the session discussions and exercise to help them with the assignment.

Participants should keep their completed assignments in their session logs filed under the appropriate session. Answer any questions but do not influence ratings.

During assignment completion time, draw a table on the flip chart, as shown below. After participants have completed their assignment, ask them to read out their statements and note them on the flip chart. Facilitate group discussion of results.

Someone to watch over me

Assignment Table 1 Someone to watch over me

	Participant 1	Participant 2	Participant 3	Participant 4
ACTIVATING EVENT				
AUTOMATIC THOUGHTS				
RULE				
DID YOUR WATCHING SELF TALK TO YOU?				
OUTCOME				
EMOTIONAL CONSEQUENCE				

3 Complete evaluation questionnaire [20 minutes]

Ask participants to complete the feedback questionnaire. Answer any questions but do not influence ratings. Questions relating to activities of daily and community living will begin to be relevant as from this session. However, participants may still give these negative ratings. Reassure them by telling them that it is perfectly acceptable to disagree with some of the statements of the questionnaire. Collect the questionnaires upon completion.

Notes

1 Take notes of all proceedings during the session including the contents of the flip chart. At the end of the session collect all materials and documents and hand them to the group practitioner well before the next group session.

2 Alternatively, you could photocopy participants' assignment tables, combine them and hand them to the practitioner.

3 Take notes of all proceedings during the session including the contents of the flip chart. At the end of the session collect all material and documents and hand them to the group practitioner well before the next group session.

4 Take notes of all proceedings during the session including the contents of the flip chart. At the end of the session collect all material and documents and hand them to the group practitioner well before the next group session.

5 Take notes of all proceedings during the session including the contents of the flip chart. At the end of the session collect all material and documents and hand them to the group practitioner well before the next group session.

6 Take notes of all proceedings during the session including the contents of the flip chart. At the end of the session collect all material and documents and hand them to the group practitioner well before the next group session.

MODULE 3

Mastering change

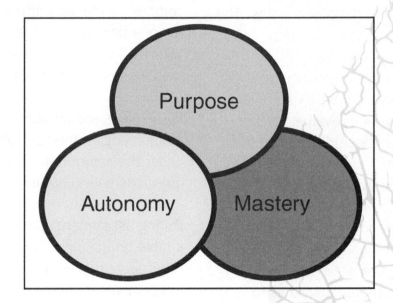

Breaking rules voluntarily

Assignment session outline[1]
1 Remember key points of the session
2 Complete assignment table
3 Complete evaluation questionnaire

1 Remember key points of the session [20 minutes]

Help/prompt participants to recall the key points of the session in their own words. The key points were:

- Automatic thoughts and consequent negative emotions occur when we construe events without evaluating the reality-base of our cognitions, perceptions and interpretations
- When we appraise events 'on-line' in this way, they may engulf us and make us feel that we might lose control
- We can develop the ability to step back and to reality-test the accuracy of our thoughts and interpretations, so as to think through critical events and evolve solutions to the problems they pose
- We can learn to recognise the Watching Self as the agent that enables us to step back from events and reality-test our cognitions and interpretations

- By visualising critical events, we learn to call up vivid images of what we need to practise in advance of real-life experiencing

2 Complete assignment table[2] [20 minutes]

Participants may need your help in completing the assignment tables despite the practice they have received during the session. Refer to the session discussions and exercise to help them with the assignment.

Participants should keep their completed assignments in their session logs filed under the appropriate session. Answer any questions but do not influence ratings.

During assignment completion time, draw a table on the flip chart, as shown below. After participants have completed their assignment, ask them to read out their statements and note them on the flip chart. Facilitate group discussion of results.

Breaking rules voluntarily

Assignment Table 1 Someone to watch over me

	Participant 1	Participant 2	Participant 3	Participant 4
RULE				
RULE-BREAK ACTIVATING EVENT				
AUTOMATIC THOUGHTS				
EXPECTED OUTCOME				
WHAT DID WATCHING SELF SAY?				
DESIRED OUTCOME CONSEQUENCE				

3 Complete evaluation questionnaire [20 minutes]

Ask participants to complete the feedback questionnaire. Answer any questions but do not influence ratings. Questions relating to activities of daily and community living will begin to be relevant as from this session. However, participants may still give these negative ratings. Reassure them by telling them that it is perfectly acceptable to disagree with some of the statements of the questionnaire. Collect the questionnaires upon completion.

Before ending this assignment session, remind participants that next week there will be a virtual reality exposure with relaxation exercise, and it would be useful for participants to bring their recording devices to capture this exercise for playback at home. Participants should also bring pillows to optimise their comfort during relaxation and a scarf with which to cover their eyes to minimise distraction.

Breaking rules voluntarily: confronting our fears, learning to be boss

Assignment session outline

1 Remember and discuss key points of the session
2 Repeat relaxation exercise in full using recording
3 Go over next week's assignment
4 Complete evaluation questionnaire

1 Remember key points of the session [20 minutes]

Help/prompt participants to recall the key points of the session in their own words. Ask them to clarify and explain.

The key points were:

The five learning points of relaxation training:

1 Reinforcement mechanism that maintains our dysfunctional rules
2 Characteristics of SMART scenarios and selection of critical events for exposure
3 Communicating whilst in a relaxed state
4 Making relaxation work
5 Developing the skills to self-relax

Feedback:

Obtain general feedback on relaxation exercise; you will obtain detailed feedback at the end of the repeat exercise

2 Repeat relaxation exercise in full using recording

This repetition has a two-fold purpose:

- Increase habituation to critical event in preparation for real-life behavioural experiment

- Practise relaxation for full rehearsal of the exercise at home

Obtain detailed feedback that compares this assignment's repeat relaxation exercise with that of the group session. Comparison feedback to cover:

- Quality of participants' relaxation and imagery
- Watching Self
- Safe place

3 Go over next week's assignment

Link this section to feedback and discuss any concerns that participants may have.

4 Complete evaluation questionnaire [20 minutes]

Ask participants to complete the feedback questionnaire. Answer any questions but do not influence ratings. Questions relating to activities of daily and community living will begin to be relevant as from this session. However, participants may still give these negative ratings. Reassure them by telling them that it is perfectly acceptable to disagree with some of the statements of the questionnaire. Collect the questionnaires upon completion.

Remind participants to bring recording devices, pillows and scarves for next week's relaxation exercise.

Are our negative beliefs about ourselves true?

Assignment session outline

1 Remember and discuss key points of the session
2 Repeat relaxation exercise in full using recording
3 Preparation to evaluate negative core beliefs
4 Go over next week's assignment
5 Complete evaluation questionnaire

1 Remember key points of the session [20 minutes]

Help/prompt participants to recall the key points of the session in their own words. Ask them to clarify and explain.

The key points were:

- Effective coping means mastery of critical events
- Repeat of the relaxation exercise with a different critical event scenario
- Comparing this session's relaxation exercise with that of the previous session and home rehearsal during feedback
- Preparing to evaluate negative core beliefs by identifying their components and rating them in light of participants' achievements in the last four sessions [Sessions 10 to 13]

2 Repeat relaxation exercise in full using recording

This repetition has a two-fold purpose:

- Increase habituation to critical event in preparation for real-life behavioural experiment
- Practise relaxation for full rehearsal of the exercise at home

Obtain detailed feedback that compares this assignment session's repeat relaxation with that of today's group session, last week's session and home rehearsal. Comparison feedback to cover:

- Quality of participants' relaxation and imagery
- Watching Self
- Safe place

3 Preparation to evaluate negative core beliefs

Review with participants their work during the group session. Specifically, go over with them their:

- Definition of their components
- Rating of these components within the context of their achievements in the last four sessions [Sessions 10 to current]

4 Go over next week's assignment

Discuss any concerns that participants may have.

5 Complete evaluation questionnaire [20 minutes]

Ask participants to complete the feedback questionnaire. Answer any questions but do not influence ratings. Questions relating to activities of daily and community living will begin to be relevant as from this session. However, participants may still give these negative ratings. Reassure them by telling them that it is perfectly acceptable to disagree with some of the statements of the questionnaire. Collect the questionnaires upon completion.

Evidence for our beliefs and our rules

Assignment session outline
1 Remember and discuss key points of the session
2 Go over next week's assignment
3 Complete evaluation questionnaire

1 Remember key points of the session [20 minutes]

Help/prompt participants to recall the key points of the session in their own words. Ask them to clarify and explain.

The key points were:

- We revisited the assignment results in the context of the goals we achieved during behavioural experiments and re-evaluated our shared negative core beliefs
- We analysed the consequences of one of our shared dysfunctional life rules

2 Go over next week's assignment [20 minutes]

Discuss any concerns that participants may have.

3 Complete evaluation questionnaire [20 minutes]

Ask participants to complete the feedback questionnaire. Answer any questions but do not influence ratings. Questions relating to activities of daily and community living will begin to be relevant as from this session. However, participants may still give these negative ratings. Reassure them by telling them that it is perfectly acceptable to disagree with some of the statements of the questionnaire. Collect the questionnaires upon completion.

Goodbye: ABI – a life-long learning experience

Assignment session outline
1 Remember and discuss key points of the session
2 Complete evaluation questionnaire

1 Remember key points of the session [20 minutes]

Help/prompt participants to recall the key points of the session in their own words. Ask them to clarify and explain.

The key points were:

- We strongly advised the group to practise relaxation and behavioural experiments on a life-long basis whenever critical events faced them
- We identified the key learning points of the programmes' three modules
- We learned to recognise self-efficacy in ourselves through our recent and lifetime achievements
- We looked at ABI as a life-long learning experience
- We said goodbye

2 Complete evaluation questionnaire [20 minutes]

Ask participants to complete the feedback questionnaire. Answer any questions but do not influence ratings. Questions relating to activities of daily and community living will begin to be relevant as from this session. However, participants may still give these negative ratings. Reassure them by telling them that it is perfectly acceptable to disagree with some of the statements of the questionnaire. Collect the questionnaires upon completion.

Notes
1 Take notes of all proceedings during the session including the contents of the flip chart. At the end of the session collect all materials and documents and hand them to the group practitioner well before the next group session.
2 The assignment table is attached to the programme notes.
3 Take notes of all proceedings during the session including the contents of the flip chart. At the end of the session collect all material and documents and hand them to the group practitioner well before the next group session.
4 Take notes of all proceedings during the session including the contents of the flip chart. At the end of the session collect all material and documents and hand them to the group practitioner well before the next group session.
5 Take notes of all proceedings during the session including the contents of the flip chart. At the end of the session collect all material and documents and hand them to the group practitioner well before the next group session.
6 Take notes of all proceedings during the session including the contents of the flip chart. At the end of the session collect all material and documents and hand them to the group practitioner well before the next group session.

Appendix

The purpose of the questionnaire below is to find out if your group experience is useful to you and how it can be further improved. Please give us your honest feedback.

Please indicate your choice by putting a cross X in either the YES or NO column. If your choice is YES, then indicate how strongly you agree by putting a circle around one of the numbers in the INTENSITY OF AGREEMENT column.

1 = Entirely Agree; 2 = Mostly Agree; 3 = Agree a Little

	Yes	Intensity of Agreement	No
1 I am more involved in community activities than I was before I started the group			
2 I manage my time better now than I did before I joined the group			
3 This session improved my understanding of myself			
4 I see more of my friends now than I did before I joined the group			
5 I like myself better now than I did before I joined the group			
6 I am more effective now in doing my household chores than I was before I started the group			
7 I enjoyed this session			
8 I get more involved with my family now than I was before I started the group			
9 This session taught me new things about myself			
10 The topics we covered were relevant to my life			
11 I can control my emotions better now than I did before I joined the group			
12 I learned new things about my brain injury in this session			
13 I think I would find the group more useful to me if . . .			

If you have selected YES to the following items, please give examples

	Examples
1 I am more involved in community activities than I was before I started the group	
2 I manage my time better now than I did before I joined the group	
4 I see more of my friends now than I did before I joined the group	
6 I am more effective now in doing my household chores than I was before I started the group	
8 I get more involved in family activities now than I did before I started the group	
11 I can control my emotions better now than I did before I joined the group	

Bibliography

Amoros, E., Martin, J.-L., and Laumo, B. (2006). Under-Reporting of Road Crash Casualties in France. *Accident Analysis and Prevention* 38: 627–635.

Bandura, A. (1977). Self-Efficacy: Toward a Unifying Theory of Behavioural Change. *Psychological Review* 84(2): 191–215. doi: 10.1037/0033–295x.84.2.191. PMID 847061

Bandura, A. (1994). Self-Efficacy. In V. S. Ramachaudran (Ed.), *Encyclopedia of Human Behaviour* (Vol. 4, pp. 71–81). New York: Academic Press. (Reprinted in H. Friedman [Ed.], *Encyclopedia of Mental Health*. San Diego: Academic Press, 1998).

Belcastro, C., and Foster, J. (2010). *Aircraft Loss-of-Control Accident Analysis*. AIAA Guidance, Navigation, and Control Conference, Guidance, Navigation, and Control and Co-Located Conferences. http://dx.doi.org/10.2514/6.2010-8004

Boyle, G. J. (1995). *Myers-Briggs Type Indicator (MBTI): Some Psychometric Limitations*. http://epublications.bond.edu.au/hss_pubs/26

Briggs, K. C., Myers-Briggs, I., and McCaulley, M. H. (1998). *Myers-Briggs Type Indicator, Form M*. Palo Alto, CA: Consulting Psychologist Press.

Briggs-Myers, I., & Briggs, K.C. (1985). *Myers-Briggs Type Indicator (MBTI)*. Palo Alto, CA: Consulting Psychologists Press.

Cicerone, K. D., and Azulay, J. (2007, September/October). Perceived Self-Efficacy and Life Satisfaction After Traumatic Brain Injury. *Journal of Head Trauma Rehabilitation* 22(5): 257–266. doi: 10.1097/01.HTR.0000290970.56130.81

Fisher, P., and Wells, A. (2009). *Metacognitive Therapy*. London: Routledge. ISBN 978-0-415-43498

Howes, R. J., and Carskadon, T. G. (1979). Test-Retest Reliabilities of the Myers-Briggs Type Indicator as a Function of Mood Changes. *Research in Psychological Type* 2(1): 67–72.

Jung, C. G. (1971). *Psychological Types. Collected Works of C.G. Jung, Volume 6*. Princeton, NJ: Princeton University Press. ISBN 0-691-097704

Kilmann, R. H., Covin, T. J., and Associates. (1988). *Corporate Transformation Revitalising Organisations for a Competitive World*. Hoboken, NJ: Jossey-Bass Publishers.

Kolb, D. (1984). *Experiential Learning as the Science of Learning and Development*. Englewood Cliffs, NJ: Prentice Hall.

Ownsworth, T., and Haslam, C. (2016). Impact of Rehabilitation on Self Concept Following Traumatic Brain Injury: An Exploratory Systematic Review of Intervention Methodology and Efficacy. *Rehabilitation* 26(1): 1–35. doi: 10.1080/09602011.2014.977924

Pittenger, D. J. (1993). Measuring the MBTI. . . and Coming Up Short. Reprinted from the Fall 1993 issue of the *Journal of Career Planning & Placement*, with permission of the College Placement Council, Inc., Copyright holder.

Pittenger, D. J. (2005). Cautionary Comments Regarding the Myers-Briggs Type Indicator. *Consulting Psychology Journal: Practice and Research* 57(3): 210–221.

Riley, G. A., Dennis, R. K., and Powell, T. (2010). Evaluation of Coping Resources and Self-Esteem as Moderators of the Relationship Between Threat Appraisals and Avoidance of Activities After Traumatic Brain Injury. *Neuropsychological Rehabilitation* 20(6): 869–882. doi: 10.1080/09602011.2010.503041

Stricker, L. J., and Ross, J. (1964). An Assessment of Some Structural Properties of the Jungian Personality Typology. *Journal of Abnormal and Social Psychology* 68: 62–71.

Teasdale, J.D., Moore, R.G., Hayhurst, H., Pope, M., Williams, S., and Segal, Z.V. (2002). Metacognitive Awareness and Prevention of Relapse in Depression: Empirical Evidence. *Journal of Consulting and Clinical Psychology* 70(2): 275–287. http://dx.doi.org/10.1037/0022-006X.70.2.275

Wells, A. (2002). *Emotional Disorders and Metacognition*. New York: John Wiley & Sons, Inc. ISBN 0-471-491691

Wells, A. (2007). Cognition About Cognition: Metacognitive Therapy and Change in Generalized Anxiety Disorder and Social Phobia. *Cognitive and Behavioural Practice* 14: 18–25.

Wells, A. (2009). *Metacognitive Therapy for Anxiety and Depression*. New York: Guilford Press. ISBN 978-1-59385-994-7

Wilson, B. A., Gracey, F., Evans, J. E., and Bateman, A. (2009). *Neuropsychological Rehabilitation*. Cambridge: Cambridge University Press. ISBN 978-0-521-84149-8

Yates, P. J. (2003). Psychological Adjustment, Social Enablement and Community Integration Following Acquired Brain Injury. *Neuropsychological Rehabilitation* 13(1): 291–306. doi: 10.1080/09602010244000408

Ylvisaker, M. (2003). Context-Sensitive Cognitive Rehabilitation After Brain Injury: Theory and Practice. *Brain Impairment* 4(1): 1–16.

Ylvisaker, M., Hanks, R., and Johnson-Greene, D. (2002). Perspectives on Rehabilitation of Individuals With Cognitive Impairment After Brain Injury: Rationale for Reconsideration of Theoretical Paradigms. *Journal of Head Trauma Rehabilitation* 17(3): 191–209.

Ylvisaker, M., Jacobs, H. E. P., and Feeney, T. (2006). Positive Supports for People Who Experience Behavioural and Cognitive Disability After Brain Injury: A Review. *Brain Impairment* 7(3): 246–258.

Young, J. E., Klosko, J. S., and Weishaar, M. E. (2003). *Schema Therapy: A Practitioner's Guide*. New York: Guilford Press.